Pandemics, Publics, and Politics

Kristian Bjørkdahl · Benedicte Carlsen
Editors

Pandemics, Publics, and Politics

Staging Responses to Public Health Crises

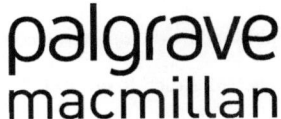

Editors
Kristian Bjørkdahl
Uni Research Rokkan Centre
Bergen, Norway

Benedicte Carlsen
Uni Research Rokkan Centre
Bergen, Norway

ISBN 978-981-13-2801-5   ISBN 978-981-13-2802-2   (eBook)
https://doi.org/10.1007/978-981-13-2802-2

Library of Congress Control Number: 2018957442

This Palgrave Pivot imprint is published by the registered company Springer Nature Singapore Pte Ltd.
The registered company address is: 152 Beach Road, #21-01/04 Gateway East, Singapore 189721, Singapore

CONTENTS

1 Introduction: Pandemics, Publics, and Politics—Staging
  Responses to Public Health Crises   1
  Kristian Bjørkdahl and Benedicte Carlsen

2 Global Health Governance and Pandemics: Uncertainty
  and Institutional Decision-Making   11
  Sudeepa Abeysinghe

3 Uncertainty and Immunity in Public Communications on
  Pandemics   29
  Mark Davis

4 Enacting Pandemics: How Health Authorities Use the
  Press—And *Vice Versa*   43
  Kristian Bjørkdahl and Benedicte Carlsen

5 "Disease Knows No Borders": Pandemics and the Politics
  of Global Health Security   59
  Antoine de Bengy Puyvallée and Sonja Kittelsen

6 When Authority Goes Viral: Digital Communication and
  Health Expertise on *pandemi.no*   75
  Kristian Bjørkdahl and Tone Druglitrø

Notes on Contributors

Sudeepa Abeysinghe is a lecturer in Global Health Policy at the University of Edinburgh. Her research focuses on the relationship between knowledge and policy in the global management of risk. She is particularly interested in the social construction of risk and uncertainty, infectious disease governance, the political sociology of institutions, and the social classification of disease.

Antoine de Bengy Puyvallée is a researcher in International Relations and research coordinator at the Center for Development and the Environment, University of Oslo. He works on global health security and the governance of global health.

Kristian Bjørkdahl is a senior researcher at Uni Research Rokkan Centre, in Bergen, Norway. His work ranges from American pragmatism to climate rhetoric, from the language of aid and humanitarianism to the rhetoric of health and medicine. He is currently working on a postdoc project about the rhetoric of Nordic colonial innocence.

Benedicte Carlsen is research leader and research professor at the Uni Research Rokkan Centre, in Bergen. She has conducted several cross-disciplinary studies within the field of science communication and implementation of scientific knowledge in professional practice. She has published extensively within her field and teaches health care students and professionals about knowledge translation.

Mark Davis is a medical sociologist with experience in clinical settings and public health research in the UK and Australia. He publishes widely on the sociology of infectious and chronic diseases, community-oriented health promotion and public health, and the narrative turns in bioethics and health communications. Mark has published widely with leading presses and journals, and written numerous reports and policy documents for government and community agencies.

Tone Druglitrø is an associate professor in science and technology studies at TIK (Centre for Technology, Innovation and Culture), University of Oslo, Norway. Her research focuses mainly on the role of non-humans in biomedical sciences and public health politics. She has published on controversies around animal experimentation, "good science," and multispecies biopolitics.

Sonja Kittelsen is a Scientia postdoctoral fellow at the Institute of Health and Society, University of Oslo. She holds a Ph.D. in International Relations from Aberystwyth University. Her current research focuses on the role of INGOs in the Global Health Security Agenda.

CHAPTER 1

Introduction: Pandemics, Publics, and Politics—Staging Responses to Public Health Crises

Kristian Bjørkdahl and Benedicte Carlsen

Abstract Pandemics are potentially very destructive phenomena, and for that reason, they both fascinate and frighten us. But because they might also turn out to be relatively mild, pandemics often become sites of contestation and conflict. Perhaps the most important characteristic of these diseases, then, is the fact that they are shot through with uncertainty. While they are only *potentially* destructive, they *necessarily* involve a great degree of uncertainty—and this is what makes the task of staging a collective response to pandemics such a challenge. In this introduction, we argue that a broader set of disciplines need to be engaged in the study of pandemics and other public health crises in order to prepare society for future pandemic events.

K. Bjørkdahl (✉) · B. Carlsen
Uni Research Rokkan Centre, Bergen, Norway
e-mail: kristian.bjorkdahl@sum.uio.no

B. Carlsen
e-mail: benedicte.carlsen@uib.no

© The Author(s) 2019
K. Bjørkdahl and B. Carlsen (eds.), *Pandemics, Publics, and Politics*,
https://doi.org/10.1007/978-981-13-2802-2_1

1

Keywords COVID-19 · Pandemics · Uncertainty · Public health

We know for certain that pandemics are potentially very destructive phenomena. The most lethal ones have with good reason become the stuff of history books. To take but one particularly ravaging example, the Spanish Flu (1918–1920) claimed somewhere between 20 and 50 million lives worldwide, and infected about a third of the planet's population—etching a sombre imprint onto our collective memory (Blakely 2006). Today, 100 years later, as we keep finding new ways to bring nature under our control, many are still concerned—and some are literally terrified—that nature might "strike back" in the form of a devastating pandemic.

Creators of fiction capitalize keenly on this fear. In recent years there has been a veritable outbreak of books and films that revolve around epidemics and pandemics—set off, perhaps, by the occurrence of an actual pandemic (the so-called "swine flu") in 2009. Book readers and movie goers have been simultaneously entertained and terrified by stories such as Steven Soderberg's film, *Contagion* (2011), Emily St. John Mandel's sci-fi novel *Station Eleven* (2014), the zombie-pandemic apocalypse, *World War Z* (2006/2013), not to mention Margaret Atwood's hugely popular *MaddAddam* trilogy (2003–2013).

Such "epidemic entertainments" (see Tomes 2002) are not, however, the only discourses that make room for our pandemic fears. In *The End of Epidemics*, medical doctor and epidemiologist, Jonathan D. Quick, provides a telling example that pandemic alarmism even thrives within medical discourse. A future pandemic "has the potential to wipe out millions of us, including my family and yours, over a matter of weeks or months," Quick writes, adding that this "looming threat to humanity" is a scenario that "makes the threat posed by ISIS [...], a ground war, a massive climate event, or even the dropping of a nuclear bomb on a major city pale by comparison" (2018: 15):

> [A] replay of the 1918 Spanish flu – against which we are not yet prepared – could hit every major city in the world within 200 days, claim more than 300 million lives, ravage national economies with the force of the Great Recession, and close public services and business around the globe. (Quick 2017)[1]

To be clear, Quick is neither an entertainer nor a creator of fiction. He is a specialist giving expert advice, and his aim is to tell us how we can improve public health preparedness around the world, so that lives that would now be lost can be saved in a future pandemic. Still, his scenarios suggest that even medical experts occasionally peddle in pandemic apocalypse.

This type of pandemic alarmism can be problematic, however. For while it is certain that pandemics *can* be very destructive, it is not certain that they *will* be so, and to stir our fears in the face of a perceived pandemic threat can all too easily turn into a situation resembling the "boy who cried wolf" (Nerlich and Koteyko 2012). To illustrate: While the seasonal influenza typically causes 290,000–650,000 respiratory deaths worldwide (WHO 2018), the death toll of the 2009 pandemic—technically termed A(H1N1)pdm09—has been estimated from 123,000 to 203,000 (Simonsen et al. 2013), making it an infinitely less destructive event than what the likes of Quick envision. In fact, many felt that the 2009 pandemic was one such that did not live up to its name. One commentator jokingly referred to as the "the little harmless Piglet virus" (Hafstad 2009).

At least in part because it turned out to become a so much milder disease than what was suggested by both authorities and media at the outbreak, the 2009 pandemic quickly became the scene of contestation—and it is far from the only such episode to have become just that. Why did the health authorities sound the alarm so violently? Were there really grounds for doing so? Who *did* sound the alarm? Was the media rather more to blame than the authorities? Did anyone have ulterior motives? What was—and what should be—the nature of the relation between the WHO, national health authorities, and the big pharmaceutical companies? Also: Might the vaccines actually be dangerous? Had the authorities in fact joined in a conspiracy with Big Pharma to drug the population?

The fact that all these questions and many more were asked during and after the 2009 pandemic, might illustrate that such episodes are shot through with uncertainty. Uncertainty, we should note, is not the same as a *threat*, nor is it equal to *fear*, though it is intimately connected with both. We can think of uncertainty as a mental and emotional space that we cannot fill using reliable methods. Our natural tendency is to fill such space, however, and in the absence of reliable methods that generates "knowledge," we proceed to fill it with all sorts of other things—hopes and fears, expectations and entitlements, scepticism and doubt.

One aspect of pandemic uncertainty concerns the disease itself. It is not necessarily clear, at any point in the course of a pandemic, how the disease will develop, what its effects will be. During the 2009 pandemic, for instance, scientific experts and other commentators worried that this mild disease might mutate, and hence present us with a much more acute predicament. It is part of the purpose of this book, however, to show that uncertainty in the face of a pandemic concerns much more than the epidemiology of the disease. While questions about how far and how fast the disease spreads, how lethal it will turn out to be, whether and how it will mutate, and so on, are real and important questions on which any serious pandemic response must rest, it would be wrong to think that these are the only questions that need answering, the only spaces of uncertainty that need filling. Rather, medical uncertainty is entangled with all sorts of other concerns that have little to do with the disease as such. It is the contention of this book that our pandemic perception and response is a messy blend of epidemiology and culture, medicine and politics, science and society.

More specifically, with the title of this volume, *Pandemics, Publics, and Politics*, we want to suggest that the epidemiology of the disease (*Pandemic*) will always be entangled with issues of public communication (*Public*), as well as with systems and practices of governance (*Politics*). To say that these entities are "entangled" is to point out that epidemiology and medical response are themselves communicative and political phenomena. Epidemiological research and monitoring do not take place in a cultural or social vacuum, but rather within particular institutions, where culturally conditioned actors perform more or less routinized practices according to the conventions of their historically contingent scientific disciplines. As far as output goes, the knowledge generated by this scientific community is literally of no use if it does not integrate with the systems of governance in place, or if it does not translate that knowledge into an idiom that lay people can understand and use.

For these reasons, we believe that preparedness in the face of pandemics requires a more sophisticated understanding of the many extra-medical facets of the disease. Among other things, we need to understand better how we tend to fill spaces of uncertainty with content that does not emanate from a scientific discourse, and which might not be what is needed in order to prepare. We need thus a broader and more heterogeneous understanding of what a "pandemic" is made up of, where that term does not simply denote a medical phenomenon which threatens human culture and society, but rather a phenomenon which, in many unpredictable ways, already *is* human culture and society. This does certainly not mean that we should disregard the role—actual or ideal—of epidemiologists. But it does mean that we should acknowledge that our capacity for pandemic response rests not on epidemiological expert knowledge alone, but also on other sorts of expertise—concerning the political systems that are designed to transform that knowledge into action, as well as concerning pandemic communication. Preparedness in the face of pandemics might even require expertise concerning "alternative expertise" or even anti-expertise movements, for how can we effectively transform medical knowledge into workable public health advice if a substantial part of the population distrusts mainstream medical knowledge?

To illustrate: Today, a case can probably be made against alarmists like Quick. A new Spanish Flu seems unlikely today, not least because medicine, and the public health apparatus, including disease prevention and control, has progressed greatly in the last 100 years. Vaccines and vaccination schemes are one obvious advance. But because pandemics are more than medical phenomena, it is uncertain how great our advances have really been. To be certain that we are now in a better position to respond to a pandemic, we would have to have made advances in our knowledge of communication and politics that could match those we have made within epidemiology.

To put it plainly, we need not just to know the new virus that emerges, but also what new forms of communication and social interaction that have emerged since the last comparable crisis. We might illustrate this by the simple fact that, since the latest pandemic, the use of social media has gone up, while the reading of traditional newspapers (and viewing of TV news) has gone down. What does it mean for a pandemic response that news is now in 2.0 mode? A whole host of sub-questions emerge: How does the so-called "#republic" (Sunstein 2017) create new conditions in which to communicate science advice in a situation of pandemic (or similar) crisis? Where has the recent spike in vaccine skepticism come from, and how can it be countered? How does one establish credibility as epidemiological expert in a situation where an increasing number of people entertain the idea that pandemics are a conspiracy concocted by the health authorities?

These are just some of the questions that stand out as essential, both in their own right and for the practical purpose of pandemic preparedness and response. The chapters of this book can only begin to answer some of them, and there will be much left to do. The point, however, is that if we open up the study of pandemics and pandemic response to new fields of—humanities and social science—research, we need to do so constantly, in an effort to understand how the society that constantly emerges brings with it a new set of conditions for our responsive capacity. To put it differently, a pandemic becomes a pandemic only because the disease is new, but culture and politics moves at least as fast as nature, so that, by the time a new disease looms, we do not just have a new disease to deal with, we also have to deal with the new society that has emerged since the previous pandemic. And while medical science has ways of monitoring, identifying, and responding to new viruses, we have no corresponding method for public communication or for politics. In these fields, we cannot predict the future and we are typically not in "control." This makes the ambition to learn from pandemics exceedingly difficult. To expect, argue Craddock and Giles-Vernick, that we by studying past pandemics can arrive at "a list of easy steps to follow for current and future preparedness plans or intervention measures," would be "detrimental in its simplicity and overgeneralization" (2010: 2). This is not just, as they acknowledge, because "both history and pandemics are complex" (2010: 2), but because we never know where societal change will take us, and hence, what type of Publics and Politics we need to prepare for.

There is already a great deal of research done on pandemic response, and our body of knowledge is constantly being supplemented. The ownership to this object of study, however, is somewhat skewed. The great majority of research being done on pandemics is done by medical researchers or public health scholars. To some extent, this is obviously how things have to be. Pandemics are medical phenomena. But if we are right to suggest that they are *also* communicative and political phenomena, the issue of pandemics and pandemic response should attract the attention of a much broader range of scholarship.

Not only can pandemics and other public health crises be an interesting object of study for humanists and social scientists, but these researchers' areas of expertise are at the heart of our ability to understand and respond to such episodes. To see pandemics as entangled clusters of diseases, publics, and politics, is to take an interest in the particularities of *how we live now*. Pandemics and pandemic response alike are the products of practices of particular times and places, and we face an imperative to tackle the distinctive features that create and condition such episodes at each time and place. Today, these include such factors as the fragmentation of media, tribalization of "knowledge regimes," the increasingly troubled status of scientific and political authority, growing cross-continental mobility, as well as the globalization, commercialization, and securitization of pandemic response systems. The central questions of this book are thus: What difference do the distinctive complexities of our day make for our ability to enact appropriate pandemic response? And how can those complexities best be studied and handled?

*

In Chapter 2, "Global Health Governance and Pandemics: Uncertainty and Institutional Decision-Making," sociologist **Sudeepa Abeysinghe** shows how pandemic events require the complex architecture of global health governance to demonstrate cohesion and efficacy. She provides an example of how the WHO sought to meet this challenge during the 2009 influenza pandemic, examining the organization's role in informing and coordinating diverse global health actors, and the tensions inherent in acting swiftly and effectively in managing a pandemic. For the WHO, Abeysinghe argues, this involved both making decisions in the face of emerging and incomplete evidence and balancing the demands of competing actors. The reward for this balancing act was not always grateful: Among other reactions, the WHO met accusations that the organization had "manufactured" the pandemic, by exaggerating the risk posed by the event.

In Chapter 3, "Uncertainty and Immunity in Public Communications on Pandemics," sociologist **Mark Davis** examines uncertainty in the expert advice on pandemics given to the general public. The chapter draws on research conducted in Australia and Scotland on public engagements with the 2009 influenza pandemic and discusses implications for communications on more recent infectious disease outbreaks, including Ebola and Zika. Davis shows how public health messages aim to achieve a workable balance of warning and reassurance and deflect problems of trust in experts and science. He further considers how uncertainties which prevail in pandemics reinforce the personalization of responses to pandemic risk, in ways that undermine the cooperation and collective action which are also needed to respond effectively to pandemics.

In Chapter 4, "Enacting Pandemics: How Health Authorities Use the Press—And Vice Versa," rhetorical scholar **Kristian Bjørkdahl** and social anthropologist **Benedicte Carlsen** point out that pandemics and other public health crises typically become big news stories, but that not much is known about the dynamics that make them so. In an interview-based study of health authorities and newspaper editors in Norway, Bjørkdahl and Carlsen explore how the dynamics between these two sets of actors contributed to the mediation of the 2009 pandemic. They find that these actors made assumptions about the other party that did not match that party's understanding of itself. The authorities, in particular, relied on a communications strategy that made unrealistic—even wrong—assumptions about how the media work, and this caused a need to back-track, and adjust their communication, and also, very likely, uncertainty and even confusion in the public as to the seriousness of the disease.

In Chapter 5, "'Disease Knows No Borders': Pandemics and the Politics of Global Health Security," international relations scholars **Antoine de Bengy Puyvallée** and **Sonja Kittelsen**, argue that the threat of a pandemic has gained prominence on policymakers' agendas due to the emergence and resurgence of infectious diseases and an increasingly interconnected world. Encapsulated by the phrase "disease knows no borders," this new risk environment has led to the rise of a new global health security regime, codified in the 2005 International Health Regulations and based on a paradigm of rapid detection and response to outbreak events, and a norm of collective action. Drawing on examples from the 2014–2015 Ebola epidemic, Puyvallée and Kittelsen argue that pandemic preparedness is not just a technical matter, but also a political and normative one. The authors show that the global health security regime carries tensions that reflect asymmetries in actors' capacities to put forward their priorities.

In Chapter 6, "When Authority Goes Viral: Digital Communication and Health Expertise on *pandemi.no*," rhetorical scholar **Kristian Bjørkdahl** and STS scholar **Tone Druglitrø** point out that our understanding and use of digital media is undoubtedly going to be a central aspect of pandemic preparedness in the future. It is still too soon to say exactly how the authorities will take advantage of the "affordances" of digital media, but one sensible assumption is that these media will create new conditions for how the authorities can establish their authority vis-à-vis the public. Bjørkdahl and Druglitrø use the Norwegian government's 2009 pandemic website, *pandemi.no*, as a case, and study its ways of establishing authority through its use of the website's various material possibilities. Arguing that the site somewhat paradoxically rests in a strikingly traditional conception of health expertise, Bjørkdahl and Druglitrø reflect on how the materiality of digital media can and should be used to communicate about pandemics in the future.

Note

1. Jonathan D. Quick, "Why I Wrote *The End of Epidemics*," 28 November 2017. https://www.msh.org/blog/2017/11/28/why-i-wrote-the-end-of-epidemics.

References

Blakely, Debra. 2006. *Mass Mediated Disease: A Case Study Analysis of Three Flu Pandemics and Public Health Policy*. Lanham: Lexington Books.

Giles-Vernick, Tamara, Susan Craddock, with Jennifer Gunn. 2010. *Influenza and Public Health: Learning from Past Pandemics*. London: Earthscan.

Hafstad, Anne. 2009. Hva skal vi tro? *Aftenposten*, 31 October, p. 3.

Nerlich, Brigitte, and Nelya Koteyko. 2012. Crying Wolf? Biosecurity and Metacommunication in the Context of the 2009 Swine Flu Pandemic. *Health & Place* 18 (4): 710–717.

Quick, Jonathan D. 2017. Why I Wrote *The End of Epidemics*, 28 November. https://www.msh.org/blog/2017/11/28/why-i-wrote-the-end-of-epidemics.

Quick, Jonathan D. 2018. *The End of Epidemics: The Looming Threat to Humanity and How to Stop It*. New York: St. Martin's Press.

Simonsen, Lone, Peter Spreeuwenberg, Roger Lustig, Robert J. Taylor, Douglas M. Fleming, Madelon Kroneman, Maria D. Van Kerkhove, Anthony W. Mounts, W. John Paget, The GLaMOR Collaborating Teams. 2013. Global Mortality Estimates for the 2009 Influenza Pandemic from the GLaMOR Project: A Modeling Study. *PLoS Medicine* 10 (11): e1001558. https://doi.org/10.1371/journal.pmed.1001558.

Sunstein, Cass. 2017. *#Republic: Divided Democracy in the Age of Social Media*. Princeton: Princeton University Press.

Tomes, Nancy. 2002. Epidemic Entertainments: Disease and Popular Culture Early-Twentieth-Century America. *American Literary History* 14 (4): 625–652.

WHO. 2018. Influenza (Seasonal). WHO Fact Sheet. http://www.who.int/mediacentre/factsheets/fs211/en/.

CHAPTER 2

Global Health Governance and Pandemics: Uncertainty and Institutional Decision-Making

Sudeepa Abeysinghe

Abstract Because novel strains of influenza can spread quickly across the globe, they require swift decision-making, often in the absence of complete or unambiguous evidence. Such disease also necessitates the coordination of multiple actors, whose interests are not always aligned. Pandemic events therefore place pressure on the cohesion and efficacy of the complex architecture of global health governance. This chapter assesses the global health management of the 2009 pandemic, focusing especially on the actions and criticisms of the World Health Organization (WHO), and assessing the strengths and limitations of the WHO's pandemic management process. The chapter highlights the difficulties involved in reacting to an evolving and uncertain risk, and situates the problem of uncertainty within the context of shifts in the WHO's institutional role within global health governance.

S. Abeysinghe (✉)
University of Edinburgh, Edinburgh, UK
e-mail: sudeepa.abeysinghe@ed.ac.uk

© The Author(s) 2019
K. Bjørkdahl and B. Carlsen (eds.), *Pandemics, Publics, and Politics*,
https://doi.org/10.1007/978-981-13-2802-2_2

11

Keywords COVID-19 · H1N1 · 2009 pandemic · Risk · Uncertainty · Institutions · Governance · WHO · Contestation

Severe epidemic and pandemic threats are potentially catastrophic. With increasing globalization, risk management needs to be undertaken at the global level. Understanding risk management as a problem of global health governance is therefore key to appreciating contemporary action surrounding infectious disease. Managing crises through the structures of global health can be challenging in several ways. Emerging and reemerging diseases are often novel (e.g. new strains of virus or bacteria) and/or poorly understood. Even during events where many of the scientific aspects of the disease are well-known (e.g. the West Africa Ebola outbreak of 2014), institutional, social, cultural and political contexts differ. Further, when considering globalised threats, multiple actors and interests must be represented and weighed against each other. These complexities are evident when focusing on the case of the WHO's management of A(H1N1)pdm09—i.e. the 2009 pandemic.

The WHO provides information and coordinates global reactions to influenza pandemics. In the past, the WHO had been more directive in its authority of epidemic disease, for example, in the malaria or tuberculosis control campaigns (Beigbeder 1998; Fee et al. 2008). Under the International Health Regulations (IHR) (2005) the WHO is pivotal in the initial definition of pandemic events, effectively serving to categorise a threat as a pandemic. This act of definition is bound by classificatory mechanisms (through application of the 2009 Pandemic Alert Phases) which trigger a public health response. Though most epidemic events can be easily distinguished, in some cases the construction of the event is fragile and unstable, lending to contestation. In such cases, the assumptions behind the phenomenon unravel. Prior to H1N1, it was generally assumed by key scientific and institutional stakeholders (including the WHO itself) that a pandemic event could be easily identified (Doshi 2011). This chapter will show that, up until H1N1 the status of a pandemic event was taken for granted. What H1N1 and the WHO's response did was to expose the fragility of the pandemic as a scientific fact. Following this, not only was the management of the threat called into question, but also the WHO's authority (Abeysinghe 2017).

The following analysis is drawn from broader work which used qualitative document analysis of texts produced by the WHO and the Council of Europe to examine the construction and subsequent contestation of the 2009 pandemic. This included all publicly available H1N1-related WHO documents such as situation updates, Director-General Speeches and Statements, Pandemic briefing notes, press briefings and key policy documents. Council of Europe documents included the tabled motion "Faked Pandemics: A Threat to Public Health" (2009), transcripts and documents related to several key committees and parliamentary sittings to debate the issue, and the final report "The Handling of the H1N1 Pandemic: More Transparency Needed" (2010). These texts were assessed through thematic coding and discourse analysis (see also Abeysinghe 2016). The chapter captures a particular point in time in respect to the WHO's actions. Indeed, the experience of H1N1 resulted in shifts in many of the organisation's pandemic management processes (most notably in terms of the inclusion of measures of severity in official definitions) (Fineberg 2014). However, assessing the debate around the WHO's management of H1N1 both sheds light on those events but also illuminates the wider nature of the institutional governance of disease risk. In this chapter, I will argue that the instability of the fact of the pandemic was a result of the embedded uncertainty surrounding H1N1, the lack of pre-existing clarity surrounding the concept of pandemic, and the positioning of the WHO within global public health.

Governing Global Health Risk

In addition to issues of global health governance, I will argue that this case study reflects aspects of the transition between *normal* science and a *post-normal* form of managing risk. A key problem of H1N1 is the problem of the construction and management of risk. Normal science surrounding risk, following Kuhn (1970), is conducted by disciplinary-bound scientists, producing knowledge about a problem of their own construction. This knowledge is transformed into a stable and consistent set of facts, having undergone scientific closure (Latour and Woolgar 1979). According to this theory, where institutions can rely upon a stable understanding of risk and can impose taken-for-granted management strategies (such as, with influenza, the use of mass vaccination), they are effectively acting within this mode of risk knowledge. While normal science is also incomplete, the problems of this mode of science can generally be (thought) solvable by scientific advances, and the knowledge surrounding these risks is often relatively stable.

In contrast, forms of knowledge that are strongly contextualised where "discovery, application and use are closely integrated" (Gibbons et al. 1994: 46), result in a different orientation to risk. Under these conditions, the evidence produced is itself uncertain and often contradictory. This is because, as in the case of H1N1, the epidemiological evidence (and, to a lesser extent, virological evidence) unfolds at a timescale that is slower than that of policymaking needs. This post-normal form of science is particularly relevant when assessing policy production surrounding risks, where "the facts are inevitably uncertain, the values in dispute" (Ravetz 2004: 351) and the responsible institution must be concerned with "the management of a reality that has irreducible complexities and uncertainties" (Funtowicz and Ravetz 1994: 1882). All pandemic strains are previously unexperienced strains of influenza. The limited knowledge around novel disease is combined with the future orientation of the risk. This means that early decisions must be made to prevent a more severe crisis. In addition, the emerging knowledge base produces diverse explanations of the problem and thereby a diverse choice of policy reactions.

This wider problem of definitional uncertainty is coupled with the complexity of the governance of globalised infectious disease. As seen in the case of H1N1, divisions of authority between global and state actors (i.e. WHO and national governments) are often ambiguous (Miller 2004), leading to misunderstandings around roles and jurisdiction (Szlezak et al. 2010). The IHR does separate the roles of the WHO (coordination and provision of information) and national governments (reporting to the WHO and managing disease control at the national level). However, the erosion of the jurisdiction of the nation state, and the rise of health problems which transgress national boundaries, leaves authority over globalised public health risk indefinite (Szlezak et al. 2010; Taylor 2005). As opposed to older international models of public health, within global health governance the WHO now presents itself as primarily concerned with the coordination and facilitation of dialogue among various global public policy networks, which include not only state actors but also corporations, NGOs and other elements of civil society. Thus, although some have suggested that increasing interdependence strengthens the role of organisations such as the WHO (particularly due to their perceived neutrality) (Taylor 2005; Walt 1988), there has arguably been an overall weakening of authority, whereby the WHO has been relegated to a facilitator rather than a leader. Diverse actors within global health, including in this case pharmaceutical corporations, are treated as partners (Buse and Walt 2000; Ollila 2005). This also acted as a source of tension surrounding the WHO's actions around H1N1.

H1N1 AND THE WORLD HEALTH ORGANIZATION

The designation of a pandemic threat relies on a number of seemingly well-defined and unproblematic characteristics. Prior to the H1N1 case, these aspects were taken by the WHO to be objectively observable and/or quantifiable. However, these components of definition can all to some extent be made fragile and tenuous. As the H1N1 pandemic (and the controversy surrounding it) developed, the concept of pandemic itself was re-problematised and the terms of definition became destabilised. A key early point in the construction of this event was the act of defining the spread of H1N1 as a pandemic.

Prior to the controversy around the handling of H1N1, the concept of pandemic was treated by the WHO (and other key actors) as relatively unproblematic (Abeysinghe 2013; Doshi 2011). In defining H1N1 as a pandemic case the WHO narrative necessarily linked the virus with the broader concept of pandemic. In the early stages of the event, the WHO assumed that any pandemic (including H1N1) would result in severe health consequences. Key aspects of pandemic disease were empha-sised in making this case. These were: the novelty of the viral agent, the unpredictability of the virus, the ability for the virus to spread geograph-ically, the ability for the virus to mutate into different forms, the mass susceptibility of global populations to the virus, and lastly, a differentia-tion between "pandemic" and seasonal influenza (Abeysinghe 2013).

Of these, it seems the issue of geographical spread was key to both the narrative accounts given by the WHO representatives and the under-pinning classificatory documentation of the Pandemic Alert Phases. For example, it was asserted by the WHO that a broad (global) geographical spread is a characterising feature of a pandemic. Thus, for example, Keiji Fukuda (Special Advisor to the WHO Director-General on Pandemic Influenza) focused on issues of novelty and spread in suggesting that:

> An easy way to think about pandemic – and actually a way I have some-times described in the past – is to say: a pandemic is a global outbreak. Then you might ask yourself "What is a global outbreak?" Global outbreak means that we see both spread of the agent – and in this case we see this

new A(H1N1) virus to most parts of the world – and then we see disease activities in addition to the spread of the virus. (Fukuda 2009, 26 May)

The ability to spread quickly was therefore assumed to be a notable characteristic of pandemic influenza, and disease activities are presumed to be a function of spread. Thus it was suggested that "[i]nfluenza pandemics must be taken seriously precisely because of their capacity to spread rapidly to every country in the world" (Chan [WHO Director-General] 2009, 29 April). The global spread of a pandemic strain served as evidence warranting concern over the threat.

These notions of spread and novelty are linked with constructions of risk around assertions of the unpredictable nature of the virus. The then WHO Director-General, Margaret Chan asserted that:

> Influenza viruses are the ultimate moving target. Their behaviour is notoriously unpredictable. The behaviour of pandemics is as unpredictable as the viruses that cause them. No one can say how the present situation will evolve. (Chan 2009a, 11 June)

This emphasis on unpredictability also highlights the uncertainty experienced by the WHO itself, where the future form of the disease was unknowable yet still needed to be predictively managed. The novelty of the virus also distinguishes the pandemic case from seasonal influenza, where:

> ...the reason we are paying so much attention to this virus though, is that seasonal influenza viruses have been around the world and have been circulating for many years. And so we understand their behaviour and we know that most people... have some immunity to them; that is what makes them seasonal influenza viruses. But we also know that when a new influenza virus enters the human population, and people do not have immunity to this virus, then the levels of serious illness and the levels of deaths can be higher... (Fukuda 2009, 5 May)

Here, novelty and unpredictability are distinguishing characteristics of pandemic strains, helping to contrast pandemic influenza from seasonal flu.

However, the WHO's explanation of the difference between H1N1 and seasonal influenza—which went at the heart of the characterisation of H1N1 as a pandemic—was often unconvincing (Abeysinghe 2013).

Even during the early months, the discussions of symptomology and differences between H1N1 and seasonal flu were unclear:

> In terms of the illness itself, in the people who are developing generally milder illness, this is similar to the kinds of influenza-like illnesses that we see, so this is typically people developing fever, cough, body aches, headaches, and this is generally in keeping with what the milder spectrum of illness is. (Fukuda 2009, 5 May)

Over time, it became increasingly evident that the H1N1 pandemic would not result in large-scale excess morbidity and mortality. The distinctions between H1N1 and seasonal flu became blurred. This was particularly problematic given the widespread (although arguably inaccurate) public perception of "the flu" as a routine and often mild event (Helman 1978; McCombie 1999). That failure to distinguish between seasonal and pandemic influenza—and therefore justify the public health focus on H1N1—is symptomatic of a more fundamental weakness in the construction and communication of H1N1. This was the neglect of the dimension of severity.

In addition to the controversy surrounding the use of vaccines, competing assertions of severity versus mildness were a primary site of contestation amongst global actors, as evidenced within press conferences and meetings. Throughout the course of the pandemic, the WHO moved from a naïve and unproblematic use of the term severity towards a series of redefinitions than increasingly complexified the term. In the early texts it was evident that the WHO placed an emphasis on the importance of determining severity:

> The other question that has come to WHO is: "Is severity important?" Of course severity is important. The whole reason why we take action against diseases is because they harm people. If diseases are relatively mild, like colds, then we take certain kinds of precautions, if diseases are very severe, such as avian influenza or HIV, then we take another level of precautions. Clearly severity is an important concept for public health and how we deal with these issues. (Fukuda 2009, 26 May)

Here, severity was suggested to be a fundamental characteristic which defined the risk posed to a population by a pandemic. In the early usage, it was clear that the interest in H1N1 as a threat stemmed from its probable ability to produce severe disease—the potential severity characterised H1N1 as a risk.

However, the pandemic failed to manifest as severe in terms of global morbidity and mortality, this characterisation became increasingly untenable. The linking of severity and risk was increasingly disassociated. This occurred through a redefinition both of the term severity and of the (previously) implied correlation between severity and risk. Though many features of H1N1 mirrored seasonal flu, those which distinguished the pandemic state were highlighted here:

> …we understand that this disease is mild in the majority of cases, however, we will have some serious cases, mostly in people with underlying conditions, which is close to the pattern we see in seasonal influenza, but we can expect also some cases in people, previously healthy, who will suffer from this virus directly. (Briand [WHO Global Influenza Programme Director] 2009, 8 May)

In addition, there were renegotiations of the meaning of severity, here in suggesting that severity (rather than a stable aspect of the disease) can be mutable over time and place:

> …we have good reason to believe that this pandemic, at least in its early days, will be of moderate severity. As we know from experience, severity can vary, depending on many factors, from one country to another. (Chan 2009, 17 June)

And finally, movements towards minimising the focus on severity:

> When you think about severity, you have at least three problems....The first is defining what you mean by severity. So, are you talking about mortality? Are you talking about morbidity, or illness? Are you talking about some combination of the numbers and the severity in meaning 'severity'? What do you really mean by it?…

> Second challenge is, how do you measure it? Not simply in theory – but how do you measure it practically and in real time, in a way that can be used to inform your decisions?

> And third, how do you account for the variety in severity in different settings at the same time? So you may have a country experiencing a degree of severity very different to another…or within a country, you may have

sub-populations experiencing degrees in severity very different to the other [populations]. (Fineberg [Chair of the International Health Regulations Committee] 2010, 14 April)

It is clear therefore that the WHO faced great difficulty in mobilising an effective discourse of severity, and therefore, risk. As a result, by the final stages of the pandemic, attempts were actually made by the WHO to abandon the concept of severity altogether, by suggesting that severity is an ambiguous and meaningless term. However, given that social experiences and understandings of the term pandemic' assume that a pandemic disease will be a severe disease (Barry 2004; Herzlich and Pierret 1987; Wald 2008), this added to the instability of the institutional construction and representation of the event.

This problem was magnified by the institutional process through which the WHO handles the definition of global infectious disease events. The Pandemic Alert Phases (outlining the stages in declaring and handling a pandemic) found in the WHO's core document regarding influenza management, the *Pandemic Influenza Preparedness and Response* (2009) guidance document, had been updated just prior to the first recorded incidence of H1N1. In approaching H1N1, member states were confused and reacted with criticism to the WHO's conceptualisation of the Pandemic Phases. From the early stages of the H1N1 threat, there was an intense level of scrutiny surrounding the Phases, both in terms of the WHO's categories and in the context of the Organisation's timing of Phase increases. In addition to the consternation surrounding the 2009 redefinitions, the practical implications of the Phases produced misunderstanding; the WHO and its wider audience (particularly member states) adopted differing interpretations of the implications of the Phase categories.

During the early stages of the threat, the WHO was criticised for not acting quickly enough in moving H1N1 through the Phases. The failure of the Phases as a classificatory scheme is reinforced through an exchange where a journalist (David Brown, *Washington Post*) questions why the pandemic has not been declared since, by the WHO's own definitions, the situation appears to warrant it. In this exchange, Brown asks:

...if you could please address the question of why there seems to be so much reluctance on going to Phase 6? It is a very clear definition. The point was made, you know, long ago, that it does not measure severity.

What is to be lost by saying that it is community spreading, in the community and more than one place – which it obviously is – more than one region, we are going to go to Phase 6 and it is a mild Phase 6. Why not just bite the bullet? (Fukuda 2009, 26 May)

In response, Keiji Fukuda (WHO Special Advisor on Pandemic Influenza and Assistant Director-General) asserted that:

The answer to that is really almost another question which is: "what is to be gained by going to another Phase?"....Right now, when we look at the request: "Why cannot WHO look at going to Phase 6" coming from the countries.... And so, behind that question is the sense that many countries are already doing things that are necessary right now to address the situation. But if you go and declare Phase 6 without very clear evidence that there is a sort of change in the global situation, it can lead to extra work for countries without much gain, it can lead to some level of panic, it can lead to some level of cynicism that something is being declared but which is not usefully producing something in terms of public health benefit and gain. (Fukuda 2009, 26 May)

This quote indicates that, even at the pre-declaration stage of the event, the WHO attempted to minimise potential criticisms of prematurely/unnecessarily calling a pandemic. This was despite that fact that WHO guidelines themselves suggested that the widespread and novelty of H1N1 defined it as a pandemic strain almost immediately following discovery (Cohen and Enserink 2009). The WHO was put in this position due to the incongruity of the Phase classifications in relation to the social understanding of pandemic.

At the other end of the event, the WHO was criticised for over-extending the pandemic period and in some cases for having called the spread of H1N1 a pandemic at all (a question that will be addressed in the section below). The Phases revolve around the issue of geographical spread:

At the WHA [World Health Assembly 2009], what the countries raised was a concern and they said that currently the criteria from going to 5 and 6 are based on geographical spread, and this is true. (Fukuda 2009, 22 May)

However, the spread of disease (including mildly symptomatic or asymptomatic infection) is not necessarily directly correlated with high risk.

As the discussion regarding the Phases and severity unfolded, differences in the perception and definition of these terms became increasingly clear:

> ...what the countries said is that we are in the mixed situation and we are concerned that if we go into Phase 6 the message to our populations will be: "You should be very afraid", whereas in fact we [the WHO] think that it indicated that the virus is spreading out but the level of fear should not go up and there should not be an increase in anxiety. (Fukuda 2009, 22 May)

Subsequent to the experience of H1N1, the problem of severity is now more closely incorporated into WHO standards for defining a pandemic event. However, in terms of H1N1, this neglect of severity in the formal mechanisms for managing the disease was a fundamental weakness of the construction of the problem of H1N1.

Implications of the WHO's Construction of H1N1

After a risk is constructed, a solution must be presented. A critical part of the WHO's institutional management of the H1N1 pandemic risk was their recommendation of preventative strategies. The Organisation emphasised the importance of vaccinations. By referring to their historical utility and efficacy, vaccines were represented by the WHO as fundamental to prevention. Contemporary responses to risk often result in a (sometimes arbitrary) choice from amongst a plurality of management strategies. H1N1 occurred not only under conditions of technical and scientific uncertainty, but also under specific institutional circumstances. Policymakers tend to simplify and perceive problems in ways that limit the perceived scope of potential solutions (Janes and Corbett 2009). Given the inherent scientific uncertainty embedded within the problem of H1N1, institutional history with mass vaccination may have helped to determine the course of action.

Historically, the WHO has turned to mass immunisation campaigns as a reaction to global public health disasters. It is therefore unsurprising that immunisation was forwarded as an effective strategy against H1N1, despite (or in fact given) the under-evidenced nature of the problem. It was suggested that "all countries will need access to vaccines" (Fukuda 2009, 24 September) to effectively deal with H1N1. From the initial discovery of the viral spread, vaccinations were focused upon as a valuable reaction. As the WHO put it:

Why are we so interested in vaccines against this new virus? It is because we all know that vaccines are an extremely effective public health tool and in addition, vaccines against seasonal influenza are protective against the disease – in severe disease – of millions of people every year. So, therefore, it is generally recognized and accepted that it would be critically important to have a vaccine if you want to stop the pandemic that might be coming with this virus. (Fukuda 2009, 1 May)

Vaccinations were therefore strongly advocated as the most effective method of minimising the risk of H1N1 in the WHO's perspective on the pandemic. The efficacy and safety of vaccines was highlighted and key work was performed in coordinating the production and supply of vaccines.

This emphasis on mass vaccination was a key site of contestation of the actions of the WHO. The Council of Europe's interest in the WHO's handling of H1N1 began at the end of 2009. One of the loudest voices of criticism of the actions of the WHO came from the German epidemiologist and Council of Europe parliamentarian Wolfgang Wodarg. This was the first institutional critic of the WHO's handling of H1N1. Wodarg presented a recommendation, endorsed by thirteen other members, to the Council on the 18th of December 2009 entitled "Faked Pandemics: A Threat to Public Health". The motion suggested that:

In order to promote their patented drugs and vaccines against flu, pharmaceutical companies have influenced scientists and official agencies, responsible for public health standards, to alarm governments worldwide. They have made them squander tight health care resources for inefficient vaccine strategies and needlessly exposed millions of people's health to the risk of unknown side-effects of insufficiently tested vaccines. ...

The definition of an alarming pandemic must not be under the influence of drug-sellers. The member states of the Council of Europe should ask for immediate investigations in the consequences at national as well as European levels. (Wodarg 2009, 18 December)

This motion foreshadowed what would become key themes in the debate surrounding the actions of the WHO, namely assertions of the undue alarm caused by the declaration of a pandemic and the inappropriate influence of the vaccine manufacturing industry upon the WHO's actions. This was all associated with the primary claim that a "true" pandemic state had not existed.

The WHO did not present either itself or its actions in a convincing manner, leaving the facts of the pandemic liable to contestation. Given that one of the WHO's primary roles in global epidemic management is in the communication of information, the failure to produce a robust narrative around H1N1 was key to the subsequent contestation. For the Council of Europe, the WHO's actions appeared not to have been supported by scientific/objective evidence. The allegedly "unscientific" actions of the WHO were presented as a key issue. For example, the Council of Europe rapporteur on the issue stated that:

> Exactly a year ago, a very bad decision was taken by the World Health Organization that now seems unscientific and irrational. The result of that decision was that the whole world became scared that a major plague was on the way – a new pandemic that would have been as bad, according to reports, as the flu pandemic of 1918. There seems to have been no scientific basis for that decision. (Flynn in Council of Europe Parliamentary Assembly 2010, 24 June)

This quote suggests that the Organisation defied scientific evidence in its decision-making process. However, the climate of scientific uncertainty under which the WHO operated rendered them susceptible to such critique after the events. The Council of Europe fundamentally contested definitions of pandemic, the legitimacy of the WHO's risk narrative surrounding H1N1, the WHO's definition of Pandemic Phase categories, and the management strategy emphasising vaccine use. In so doing, through illustrating the ineffectual construction of the H1N1 pandemic, the legitimacy and institutional processes of the WHO itself were made susceptible to critique.

More broadly, apart from direct criticisms such as those outlined above, the instability of the WHO's positioning was evident. The WHO was seen by some actors (such as in the Council of Europe's account) as a central directing body. Thus, for example, although the then-Director-General Margaret Chan appeared to take responsibility when she suggested that "[t]he decision to declare an influenza pandemic will fall on my shoulders [and] I can assure you, I will take this decision with utmost care and responsibility" (Chan 2009, 8 May). However, there is also a distinct sense in which the position of the WHO was dependent upon the actions of member states and other stakeholders such as pharmaceutical corporations. In this way, input of multiple partners was emphasised. For example, in announcing the decision to declare a pandemic, Chan suggested that Organisation had "conferred with leading influenza experts, virologists, and public health officials" (Chan 2009b, 11 June). This impression of the WHO's actions as being dependent upon and a result of the input of multiple individuals, governments and organisations was clearly distinct from the narratives of critics and commentators more generally, who tended to portray the WHO as solely responsible for making the decision to call a pandemic and dictating reaction (Wodarg 2009; Flynn 2010).

The WHO represented itself as a coordinating body which provided a source of global information. In regards to their narrative and practice of global public health, the practical implications of the blurring of the roles of various stakeholders were evident. A good illustration of these implications was the Organisation's reaction to pharmaceutical manufacturers

> ...maintaining and engaging the private manufacturing sector has been a very critical step, again, because this group has the unique and essential role in the vaccine manufacturing process....In the first place it's the private sector which makes vaccines ......Also, this group that has really a unique expertise and knowledge of vaccines because of their manufacturing of the vaccines, it's essential for public health really to act on this kind of knowledge and know-how.... (Fukuda 2009, 3 December)

The emphasis on solidarity and treating all actors as partners had important flow-on consequences. For example, throughout it was clear that the WHO emphasised "the absolute need to extend preparedness and mitigation measures to the developing world" (Chan 2009a, 11 June) and engaged in advocacy with pharmaceutical manufactures around the distribution of products. Yet, simultaneously, when faced with actions from member states that went against WHO recommendations (e.g. mass culling of pigs in Egypt, disrupting the freedom of travel of Mexican citizens) little concrete action could be taken. Thus, while the WHO was liable to the initial construction of the pandemic, and held as responsible by various critics, the organisation's role within global health governance limited the ability of the WHO to direct the results of this risk construction.

CONCLUSION

The WHO did not effectively mobilise a stable construction of the H1N1 pandemic as a public health risk. This ultimately resulted in the contestation of the WHO's actions by other global health actors. In understanding this case study, we can see that the role played by scientific and institutional uncertainty in the politics surrounding the WHO and H1N1 is critical. In the context of a novel disease, where science is still in development, the WHO needed to make policy decisions in the absence of concrete evidence. The problem of dealing with an uncertain evidence base meant that the WHO's stance towards the disease over time. As this chapter has shown, this issue was particularly evident in conversations around severity and risk. While this is an understandable tactic in the face of a shifting evidence base, it also meant that the social construction of H1N1 as a public health problem was fragile. This opened the WHO's action up to critique, as evidenced by the criticisms of actors within the Council of Europe. This was all set in a context where the WHO's institutional role within the structures of global health governance has been evolving, and where the organisation now must coordinate the interest of diverse global health stakeholders rather than directly manage infectious disease crises.

Uncertainty abounds within the global governance of many politically charged risks. Contemporary "wicked problems" such as climate change, population growth and aging, and food and water scarcity, present important similarities to the prospect of a pandemic. All are global risks of a potentially catastrophic magnitude, and all are similarly framed by contestation and an emerging evidence base. Like the WHO in respect to H1N1, global institutions and national governments are placed in a position where they are forced to act, even while scientific evidence is scarce or conflicting. Representation and social construction are fundamental to the way in which such risks are perceived and managed. As Latour (2004) put it, such risks are not "matters of fact" to be taken for granted, even though they are global "matters of concern" which must be confronted. During H1N1, the facts of the case were emerging, but the WHO needed to react to the concern within the context of this underlying uncertainty. These criticisms could perhaps not have been easily anticipated beforehand. However, a more critical reflection on the mismatches between institutional assumptions (e.g. about the geographical definitions of the pandemic label) and other constructions of the problem (e.g. a public interest in severity), combined with a more persuasive narrative of risk, may have strengthened the position on the WHO in managing the pandemic.

REFERENCES

Abeysinghe, Sudeepa. 2013. When the Spread of Disease Becomes a Global Event: The Classification of Pandemics. *Social Studies of Science* 43 (6): 905–926.

Abeysinghe, Sudeepa. 2016. *Pandemics, Science and Policy: H1N1 and the World Health Organization*. London: Palgrave Macmillan.

Abeysinghe, Sudeepa. 2017. Contesting a Pandemic: The WHO and the Council of Europe. *Science as Culture* 26 (2): 161–184.

Barry, John. 2004. *The Great Influenza: The Epic Story of the Deadliest Plague in History*. London: Penguin.

Beigbeder, Yves. 1998. *The World Health Organization*. The Hague: Martinus Nijhoff.

Buse, Kent, and Gill Walt. 2000. Global Private-Public Partnerships, Part II: What Are the Health Issues for global Governance. *Bulletin of the World Health Organisation* 78 (5): 699.

Cohen, Jon, and Martin Enserink. 2009. After Delays, WHO Agrees: The 2009 H1N1 Pandemic Has Begun. *Science* 324 (5934): 1496–1497.

Doshi, Peter. 2011. The Elusive Definition of Pandemic Influenza. *Bulletin of the World Health Organization* 89 (7): 532–538.

Fee, Elizabeth, Marcos Cueto, and Theodore Brown. 2008. WHO at 60: Snapshots from Its First Six Decades. *American Journal of Public Health* 98 (4): 630–633.

Fineberg, H.V. 2014. Pandemic Preparedness and Response—Lessons from the H1N1 Influenza of 2009. *New England Journal of Medicine* 370 (14): 1335–1342.

Funtowicz, Silvio, and Jerome Ravetz. 1994. Uncertainty, Complexity and Post-Normal Science. *Environmental Toxicology and Chemistry* 13 (12): 1881–1885.

Gibbons, Michael, Camille Limoges, Helga Nowotny, Simon Schwartzman, Peter Scott, and Martin Trow. 1994. *The New Production of Knowledge: The Dynamics of Science and Research in Contemporary Societies*. London: Sage.

Helman, Cecil. 1978. "Feed a Cold, Starve a Fever": Folk Models of Infection in an English Suburban Community, and Their Relation to Medical Treatment. *Culture, Medicine and Psychiatry* 2 (2): 107–137.

Herzlich, Claudine, and Janine Pierret. 1987. *Illness and Self in Society*. Baltimore: John Hopkins University Press.

Janes, Craig, and Kitty Corbett. 2009. Anthropology and Global Health. *Annual Review of Anthropology* 38: 167–183.

Kuhn, Thomas. 1970. *The Structure of Scientific Revolutions.* Chicago: The University of Chicago Press.

Latour, Bruno. 2004. Why Has Critique Run Out of Steam?: From Matters of Fact to Matters of Concern. *Critical Inquiry* 30: 225–248.

Latour, Bruno, and Steve Woolgar. 1979. *Laboratory Life.* Beverly Hills: Sage.

McCombie, Susan. 1999. Folk Flu and Viral Syndrome: An Anthropological Perspective. In *Anthropology in Public Health: Bridging Differences in Culture and Society,* ed. Robert Hahn, 27–43. New York: Oxford University Press.

Miller, Clark A. 2004. Climate Science and the Making of a Global Public Order. In *States of Knowledge: The Co-Production of Science and Social Order,* ed. S. Jasanoff, 46–66. London: Routledge.

Ollila, Eeva. 2005. Global Health Priorities: Priorities of the Wealthy? *Globalization and Health* 1 (6): 6–11.

Ravetz, Jerome. 2004. The Post-Normal Science of Precaution. *Futures* 36 (3): 347–357.

Szlezak, Nicole, Barry Bloom, Dean Jamison, Gerald Keusch, Catherine Michaud, Suerie Moon, and William Clark. 2010. The Global Health System: Actors, Norms and Expectations in Transition. *PLoS Medicine* 7 (1): 1–4.

Taylor, Allyn. 2005. Governing the Globalization of Public Health. *Journal of Law, Medicine & Ethics* (Fall): 500–508.

Wald, Priscilla. 2008. *Contagious: Cultures, Carriers, and the Outbreak Narrative.* Durham: Duke University Press.

Walt, Gill. 1988. Globalisation of International Health. *The Lancet* 351: 434–437.

WHO. 2009. *Pandemic Influenza Preparedness and Response: A WHO Document.* Geneva: Global Influenza Programme, World Health Organization.

Other Sources

Briand, Sylvie. 2009, 8 May. *WHO Press Briefing 08/05/09.* Available at: http://www.who.int/mediacentre/multimedia/swineflupressbriefings/en/index.html.

Chan, Margaret. 2009, 29 April. *WHO Press Briefing 29/04/09b.* Available at: http://www.who.int/mediacentre/multimedia/swineflupressbriefings/en/index.html.

Chan, Margaret. 2009, 8 May. *World Is Better Prepared for Influenza Pandemic.* Address to the ASEAN+3 Health Ministers' Special Meeting on Influenza (A)H1N1, Bangkok, Thailand. Available at: http://www.who.int/dg/speeches/2009/asean_influenza_ah1n1_20090508/en/index.html.

Chan, Margaret. 2009a, 11 June. *World Now at the Start of 2009 Influenza Pandemic* Statement to the Press by WHO Director-General. Available at: http://www.who.int/mediacentre/news/statements/2009/h1n1_pandemic_phase6_20090611/en/index.html.

Chan, Margaret. 2009b, 11 June. *WHO Press Briefing 11/06/09*. Available at: http://www.who.int/mediacentre/multimedia/swineflupressbriefings/en/index.html.

Chan, Margaret. 2009, 17 June. *WHO Welcomes Sanofi-Aventis's Donation of Vaccine*. Statement by the WHO Director-General. Available at: http://www.who.int/mediacentre/news/statements/2009/vaccine_donation_20090617/en/index.html.

Council of Europe Parliamentary Assembly. 2010, 24 June. *Verbatim Report—Twenty-Sixth Sitting of the Parliamentary Assembly of the Council of Europe*. Available at: http://assembly.coe.int/Main.asp?/Documents/Records/2010/E/10062441500.htm.

Flynn, Paul. 2010, 7 June. *The Handling of the H1N1 Pandemic: More Transparency Needed* [Doc No. 12283—Passed by the Council of Europe 2010, 24 June]. Strasbourg: Social Health and Family Affairs Committee, Council of Europe.

Fineberg, Harvey. 2010, 14 April. *WHO Press Briefing 19/05/10*. Available at: http://www.who.int/mediacentre/multimedia/swineflupressbriefings/en/index.html.

Fukuda, Keiji. 2009, 1 May. *WHO Press Briefing 01/05/09*. Available at: http://www.who.int/mediacentre/multimedia/swineflupressbriefings/en/index.html.

Fukuda, Keiji. 2009, 5 May. *WHO Press Briefing 05/05/09*. Available at: http://www.who.int/mediacentre/multimedia/swineflupressbriefings/en/index.html.

Fukuda, Keiji. 2009, 22 May. *WHO Press Briefing 26/05/09*. Available at: http://www.who.int/mediacentre/multimedia/swineflupressbriefings/en/index.html.

Fukuda, Keiji. 2009, 26 May. *WHO Press Briefing 26/05/09*. Available at: http://www.who.int/mediacentre/multimedia/swineflupressbriefings/en/index.html.

Fukuda, Keiji. 2009, 24 September. *WHO Press Briefing 26/05/09*. Available at: http://www.who.int/mediacentre/multimedia/swineflupressbriefings/en/index.html.

Fukuda, Keiji. 2009, 3 December. *WHO Press Briefing 03/12/09*. Available at: http://www.who.int/mediacentre/multimedia/swineflupressbriefings/en/index.html.

Wodarg, Wolfgang. 2009, 18 December. *Faked Pandemics— A Threat to Health*. Motion of a Recommendation by the Parliamentary Assembly of the Council of Europe Doc. 122110. Strasbourg: Council of Europe.

CHAPTER 3

Uncertainty and Immunity in Public Communications on Pandemics

Mark Davis

Abstract This chapter examines uncertainty in the expert advice on pandemics given to members of the general public. The chapter draws on research conducted in Australia and Scotland on public engagements with the 2009 influenza (swine flu) pandemic and discusses implications for communications on more recent infectious disease outbreaks, including Ebola and Zika. It shows how public health messages aim to achieve a workable balance of warning and reassurance and deflect problems of trust in experts and science. The chapter considers how uncertainties which prevail in pandemics reinforce the personalization of responses to pandemic risk, in ways that undermine the cooperation and collective action which are also needed to respond effectively to pandemics.

Keywords COVID-19 · H1N1 · 2009 pandemic · Pandemic communication · Public response · Personalization · Immunity

M. Davis (✉)
School of Social Sciences, Monash University, Clayton, VIC, Australia
e-mail: mark.davis@monash.edu

© The Author(s) 2019
K. Bjørkdahl and B. Carlsen (eds.), *Pandemics, Publics, and Politics*,
https://doi.org/10.1007/978-981-13-2802-2_3

29

Uncertainty is a central challenge for public communications on matters pandemic. Recent efforts to respond to outbreaks of infectious diseases, such as pandemic (swine flu) influenza (World Health Organization 2009), Ebola (Green 2014; World Health Organization 2014) and Zika virus (World Health Organization 2016) have been marked by the limits of what can be known ahead of time and the challenges of responding to the particular turnings of outbreaks as they happen. The 2009 pandemic influenza—the topic of research I conducted with colleagues in Australia and Scotland—is a pivotal example of this problem of responding to a pandemic in real time. The 2009 pandemic put huge strain on global, national and local health systems, affecting many individuals and especially pregnant women and people with specific vulnerabilities to respiratory infections. It was a prominent, perhaps dominant, health news story of the period. But the pandemic turned out to be nothing like as severe as it was first thought to be. Moreover, there was insufficient take-up of the H1N1 vaccine (Bone et al. 2010; Galarce et al. 2011; White et al. 2010; Yi et al. 2011) and it was observed that only minorities or small majorities reported that they intended to, or did, enact recommended social isolation to avoid transmission of the virus (Kiviniemi et al. 2011; Mitchell et al. 2011; Rubin et al. 2009; Van et al. 2010). Like the "swine flu affair" of the 1970s in the United States (Fineberg 2008), the 2009 pandemic raised questions for the public health system of how to shape public action in light of the significant uncertainties which are particular to influenza, and without jeopardizing trust in government and the scientific knowledge on which is built public policy.

Central, too, was immunity, in its medical and social senses. Immunity is not simply an object of biomedicine, it is also deeply entwined with collective life and the interrelations that come with, specifically, contagious diseases. It is also important to recognize that these issues are by no means settled; how individuals conduct themselves in relation to others in time of pandemic is a central and enduring concern for public health systems. In 2009 in the UK, for example, advertisements featured images of travellers on public transport and the following text:

> If you could see flu germs, you'd see how quickly they spread. Cold and flu germs can live on some surfaces for hours. Always carry tissues with you and use them to catch your cough or sneeze. Bin the tissue, and to kill the germs, wash your hands with soap and water, or use a sanitiser gel. This is the best way to help slow the spread of flu. Protect yourself and others (NHS Swine Flu Information).

This advice addresses responsible individuals and asks them to help limit the spread of infection. The final part of the message 'Protect yourself and others' captures the idea that an easily spread influenza virus requires significant cooperation and the internalization of the idea of action on health for the collective good, as well as for oneself. This reference to altruistic action on health indicated that the social response to the 2009 pandemic exemplified biopolitics (Rose 2007). Individuals are expected and encouraged to internalize the idea that they can take action on themselves to sustain and better their health and reproductive futures. This self-subjectification applies to the advice given to members of the general public on the 2009 influenza pandemic. In addition to the advice noted above, individuals were encouraged to arrange a network of "flu friends" who could be called upon in the case of illness, to stay abreast of developments in the media, and adopt expert advice (National Health Service 2009). Publics were also advised to stay home if they suspected they were ill and to contact NHS services online or by telephone and to not attend GP surgeries of A&E, unless instructed to do so. In this view, the communications of 2009 hailed pandemic citizenship fashioned around the imperatives of action to avoid and contain the spread of infection and to make oneself available to expert advice.

In what follows I explore pandemic communications under conditions of uncertainty, as exemplified by the 2009 influenza pandemic and its resonances with other recent contagions. As we will see, uncertainty has the effect of accentuating personalized responses to expert advice. It also sponsors communicative action figured around seeking the "just right" balance of warning and reassurance and related implications for trust in expert knowledge and authority to govern.

THE EXAMPLE OF THE 2009 PANDEMIC

The events of 2009 foregrounded many of the strengths and weaknesses of public health systems across the globe. Key among these was preparedness and capacity to cope with large scale containment strategies which were used to manage the emerging pandemic. The pandemic preparedness plans in place in 2009 required that in the early phases of the pandemic, efforts should be made to sequester infected individuals and to trace their contacts so that the spreading infection could be tracked down and curbed (World Health Organization 2011). Probably a central lesson of 2009 was that such efforts were costly and apparently ineffective. In some settings public health professionals were asked to continue this method even when they were aware that the virus was spreading quickly despite their best efforts (Waller et al. 2016).

The 2009 pandemic therefore revealed the importance of being able to quickly assess the biological characteristics and severity of the infection so as to be able to modify the application of resources. Since 2009, public health systems have attended to the development of evidence-based measures to assess seriousness and the development of local and viable responses to a global pandemic threat (Australian Department of the Prime Minister and Cabinet 2011). Pandemic preparedness, therefore, has demonstrated a marked shift away from uniformity and top-down governance towards local, evidence-based, approaches. For example, Australia's 2009 version of its preparedness plan adopted a traditional method of top-down transmission of expert knowledge and advice to publics. Government in this view was mandated to:

> Deliver consistent and accurate public messages nationwide in the event of a pandemic. Governments will make every effort to provide timely and reliable advice to the public, media, businesses and industries. (Australian Department of Health and Ageing 2008: 34)

By 2014, however, the Australian pandemic policy instrument referred to the need for public communications which were "two-way" and "listening" to publics (Australian Department of Health 2014: 63). This approach to feedback on the transmission of information was said to depend on in vivo market research, the monitoring of social media, and a Q&A website where publics can pose questions and air their opinions (Australian Department of Health 2014: 63). The policy also made reference to the need for specific and tailored messages for vulnerable groups.

However, during 2009 pandemic public communications faced significant challenges, not all of which are obviously addressed in the revised policies and their emphasis on feedback loops, market research and social media. Surveys conducted at the time of the onset of the pandemic in 2009 show that while publics largely endorsed government action on the pandemic, they underestimated risk of infection and only minorities reported that they had adopted recommended behaviours such as social isolation and coughing and sneezing etiquette (Rubin et al. 2009). The findings suggest that individuals interpreted public health advice with some scepticism. Research shows also that espoused trust in government was associated with self-reported compliance with public health advice (Lin et al. 2014; Rubin et al. 2009). As noted, populations across the globe adopted vaccination only in small proportions, insufficient to protect the entire population.

This indication of weak public engagement with the pandemic may be explained by a more general effect of risk management. It is surmised that the repetition of warnings over the last few decades—for example, HIV, BSE, Avian Influenza, hospital superbugs, SARS, H1N1, Ebola and Zika, to name a few—leads to weariness on the part of publics (Joffe 2011). Diminishment in public engagement with risk is also thought to be an effect of risk society preoccupation with the forecasting and management of risks (Giddens 1998). Public weariness can be thought of as a manufactured risk in the sense that it arises through attempts to manage risk. It is also evident that news on current risks are often framed by established patterns of meaning used to depict previous or contiguous risks (Ungar 2008). It is possible, therefore, that publics have learned to screen out global health alerts and treat media on the topic with a degree of scepticism, a perspective supported by our own (Davis et al. 2014; Davis 2017) and similar research (Hilton and Smith 2010; Holland and Blood 2012). Implied also is that repeated global health alerts coupled with some scepticism on the part of publics may lead them to fall back on personal knowledge and resources.

Public Responses

The individualization of responses to pandemic risk communications was supported by our own research. Individuals in our interviews and focus groups endorsed expert advice regarding coughing and sneezing etiquette and social isolation, but they did not think that these strategies would be viable in the long run (Davis et al. 2016). Some of our respondents did adopt forms of social isolation, but they also saw in these strategies some flaws and inadequacies. They appeared, in general, to recognize the ease with which infection could occur. For these reasons, many of the people we spoke with resorted to discourse on immunity as a means of coping with a more than likely infection. Almost absent was discourse on personal action as a means of protecting all, apart from among those with severe respiratory illness who were used to dealing with the threat of infection posed by others. Our respondents focused on matters such as the building of immunity through consumer products, rest and exercise, and spoke of the need to cultivate and educate their personal immune system, with some reference to childhood experiences of exposure to infection. Individuals seemed to accept that interaction with microbial life was inevitable and important to health and that their immune systems were shaped by their own actions. This "choice immunity" was spoken of as managing one's body and those of dependent others in ways that resonated with the well-known notion of "choice biography" which is said to characterize reflexive modernization (Beck and Beck-Gernsheim 2002).

There are other implications of this resort to choice immunity. Ed Cohen has shown how immunity is a conceptual framing of subjectivity that preceded modern day microbiology (2009). With its root in the Latin *munis*—also the root for municipal and remuneration, for example—immunity referred to the suspension of one's civic and pecuniary obligation to collective life. Cohen gave examples which include, duty, gift, tax, tribute, sacrifice, and public office (2009). Immunity suspends the "bond of requirement," but also, therefore, reinscribes it (p. 41). It always and necessarily marks the power of the social obligation it refuses, including in matters of health. As Cohen showed, microbiology, and specifically germ theory, appropriated and reconfigured the metaphor of immunity to help narrate the emerging science of cells, microbes and pathogenesis. In particular, the idea of immunity helped to explain how the immune system destroyed cells colonized by alien microbial life and bypassed uninfected cells of the body, although autoimmunity and microchimerism complicate this understanding of biological immunity (Martin 2010). Combined with germ theory, immunity operates to produce a "milieu interieur;" an imaginary of the battle with microbial invaders inside the body (Cohen 2009: 239), a metaphor which accentuates the emphasis on the individual in relation to contagious health threats. Emily Martin has made a similar point that media depictions of immunity have often referred to the war within the body (1994). It is therefore no surprise that individuals resort to the practical and metaphorical properties of immunity when they are asked to contend with the risk of pandemic influenza, which creates uncertainties over which they otherwise have very little apparent control.

These issues are reflected in consumer products, for example, the commercial marketing of probiotic foods and supplements

(Burges Watson et al. 2009; Koteyko 2009; Nerlich and Koteyko 2008), which address individual consumers in terms of "choice immunity." Probiotics also raise the idea that it is important to replace bacteria that have been killed off due to antibiotic treatment and/or the idea that "good" bacteria will outcompete illness producing bacteria. The scientific underpinning and marketing of probiotics, then, depend on a division of "good" and "friendly" bacteria from disease-producing bacteria.

Be Alert, Not Alarmed

It is against this backdrop of immunity culture that public health institutions have to shape and circulate messages on how individuals ought to conduct themselves. As with the 2009 pandemic, agencies such as the WHO, regional WHO offices, and lead national public health agencies such as the CDC and Public Health Scotland implement communication strategies and are key sources of expert commentary in worldwide news media.

A central communication challenge is how to shape messages so that they are productive of desired action on the part of members of the general public, when it cannot be known absolutely how matters will transpire. It is clear from our research with public health professionals in Australia and the UK that finding a balance of motivation and reassurance was paramount (Davis et al. 2011, 2013). In this context, public health experts were concerned that publics should be advised and asked to prepare for the pandemic but not in ways that promoted anxiety or promoted panic, as reflected in, for example, runs on supermarkets, pharmacies and clinics. This meant that messages also had to be reassuring but not in a way that led publics to ignore advice, or worse, to become complacent. As Briggs and Nichter have pointed out, pandemic messaging was carefully styled around the notion of "be alert, not alarmed" (2009). They have identified this approach as the "just right" Goldilocks method, that is, the production of alert, but not panicky, reassured, but not complacent publics. For example, in a newspaper article published on 27 April 2009, in the first few days of the pandemic alert, the Chief Health Officer of Australia was quoted to have said:

> We should be aware but I'm not overly alarmed at this point. We don't have confirmed cases in Australia but I think there will be some cases in

the future. We think the population should be alert, should be aware of travellers in their midst who have the flu. But not alarmed at this point, just aware. (Robotham and Pearlman 2009)

In this way, pandemic communications help to constitute the expert-informed, life choices of individuals. Less obvious are obligations to others which also make immunity possible, such as herd immunity and the related practice of altruistic vaccination to protect vulnerable others. It is also important to recognize that explicit reference to immunity is rarely a feature of this public health advice; it is nearly always implied.

"THE BOY WHO CRIED WOLF" AND OTHER COMMUNICATION DILEMMAS

The 2009 pandemic raised some other problems related to the eventual character of the pandemic as mild for most, but not all. As noted, the 2009 pandemic was quickly found to be less severe than early indications portended, though some groups faced elevated risks and the pattern of morbidity differed from that typical for seasonal influenza (Presanis et al. 2011). It therefore became necessary to manage the communications turn away from alert, but without the cessation of cautionary messaging and continued advice for those who did face higher risk of severe disease. Influenza is known to return, on occasion, in a second wave which has the potential to be more severe for all or some of those affected (Presanis et al. 2011). Uncertainties like these meant that it was imperative to sustain a kind of watchful, just in case, attitude, until such time as an effective vaccine became available. This particular situation of a global alert followed by revisions of preparedness and response and growing evidence of a significantly less dangerous pandemic led to new communications challenges to do with explaining to publics what was happening and how they should therefore conduct themselves. This shifting in messaging across the period of the pandemic implied "the boy who cried wolf" parable (Nerlich and Koteyko 2012), which teaches in narrative form the jeopardy of trust faced by raising a false alarm, too often.

One effect of false alarm is that it may amplify the importance of choice immunity, that is, recourse to the self-reliant management of the body as the means to contend with an uncertain health threat. Sociological perspectives on choice biography point out that under the conditions of neo-liberal economic and political order, individuals are forced to rely on themselves and their own decision-making capacities, since there is in the end, nowhere else for them to go (Beck and Beck-Gernsheim 2002). They nevertheless are bound to depend on expert advice, since no one person can be expert in all the considerations that pertain to health or any other of the major life decisions (Ungar 2003). False alarm destabilizes expert authority and leaves people doubly reliant on themselves. In this view, the tendency for individuals to fall back on their immunity is a rational response to the requirement to take action and because, in the face of the uncertainties which preside in the case of influenza, the body is one apposite arena in which people are able to exercise some control.

Our research shows also that the communication on the pandemic had the potential to divide publics according to their vulnerability, another way in which knowledge and questions played out in the 2009 pandemic. They showed awareness of the "boy who cried wolf" dilemma but also recognized the invidious situation in which public health experts found themselves. They spoke of the needless hype of the media on the pandemic, by which they meant the extent of the reporting on the progress of the pandemic (Davis and Lohm forthcoming). It is important to remember, also, that some groups and individuals were affected and profoundly so, for example, women who were pregnant in 2009. Public communications on the risk of pandemic influenza, therefore, had a schismatic quality in the sense that the mildness of the virus needed to be explained to publics, while some remained at risk. Like the universalism of pandemic preparedness, communications were also faced with the need for nuance and provisionality. This splitting of publics according to their vulnerability (Stephenson et al. 2014), was suggestive also of the coexistence of different modes of pandemic subjectivity. The "not at risk and in general unconcerned" could look upon news media and public communications as needless and hyped, particularly as the pandemic progressed. Vulnerable groups, as we have suggested (Stephenson et al. 2014), at times had trouble recognizing themselves in these messages and once they had established for themselves awareness of their immunological vulnerability, they looked upon the hype as masking what for them was a real and visceral anxiety and set of practical issues of infection control and vaccination. This schism in public engagement accentuates the sense in which people have to make up their own mind on how to act in the context of what our vulnerable interviewees suggested were confusing, mixed messages.

CONCLUSION

The communications challenges of emerging, changing pandemics are considerable. Messages have to, at first, inform publics without frightening them, but also reassure them without producing complacency. As the example of the 2009 pandemic indicates, as the infection progressed and evidence emerged of the health effects of the H1N1 virus, public health systems had to explain that the pandemic was mild, though this situation could change. They also had to embed in this more general message information for minorities that they remained at serious risk. This changing, complex message risked provoking accusations of false alarm and therefore mistrust, as has happened in previous outbreak situations (Fineberg 2008). As I argued, too, the mixing of a general message of a mild pandemic which might change with messages that also some particular kinds of people were at risk, placed vulnerable people in the difficult situation of having to identify themselves in these messages and take action when others were sceptical and unlikely to be acting to protect themselves and those around them.

When we asked people in our research to talk about H1N1 and specifically if it could be prevented, people acknowledged that infection was unlikely to be avoided and, accordingly, they were forced to reflect on the capacity of their body to cope with infection. As indicated, this resort to personal immunity was not quite the same as the science of cellular immunity discussed by Cohen and others. It more closely resembled an acceptance of the possibility of the presence of the virus in the body and fashions an arena for volitional action on the body when other forms of action seem to have less practical value, as was the case in 2009. For example, social isolation and possibly vaccination, were endorsed but by and large not extensively taken up, particularly given that the virus was in general mild and easy to catch.

Because the H1N1 virus was observed to be so easily transmitted, the resort to personal immunity had doubled value. It may be for this reason that publics endorsed expert advice to self-isolate and vaccinate, but did not do so, that is, they fended for themselves and the pandemic turned into a mild one, anyway, though not for everyone. Appeals to the collective good and altruistic vaccination on which depend public health efforts concerning pandemics, may miss the point that individuals are led to think of their personal immunity as an arena within which they can sustain themselves in the face of deeply uncertain threats which arise in communal life. If as Cohen has suggested, immunity is fused with ideas of cellular action on microbial pathogens but it is also a metaphor for freedom from obligation. It seems, then, that a key lesson from 2009 was that freedom from the dangers of infection found in personal action on immunity also implied freedom from having to act in the interest of others; the more free one is from the dangers of infection—the stronger one's immunity—the less one needs to consider the dangers which others face, particularly under conditions of uncertainty. Individualized ideas of immunity in connection with uncertainties may limit the effectiveness of public health communications on influenza pandemics and other contagious threats.

Acknowledgements This chapter is based on research funded by an Australian Research Council Discovery Project grant on pandemic influenza (DP110101081). I would like to acknowledge the assistance of my colleagues from the pandemic influenza project, Niamh Stephenson, Paul Flowers, Emily Waller, Casimir MacGregor and Davina Lohm. I am also very grateful for the time and efforts of those who participated in the interviews and focus groups for the research.

REFERENCES

Australian Department of Health. 2014. *Australian Health Management Plan for Pandemic Influenza*. Canberra: Commonwealth of Australia.

Australian Department of Health and Ageing. 2008. *Australian Health Management Plan for Pandemic Influenza: Important Information for all Australians*. Canberra: Australian Government, Department of Health and Ageing.

Australian Department of the Prime Minister and Cabinet. 2011. *National Action Plan for Human Influenza Pandemic*. Canberra: Commonwealth of Australia.

Beck, Ulrich, and Elisabeth Beck-Gernsheim. 2002. *Individualisation: Institutionalised Individualism and Its Social and Political Consequences*. London: Sage.

Bone, A., J. Guthmann, J. Nicolau, and D. Levy-Bruhl. 2010. Population and Risk Group Uptake of H1N1 Influenza Vaccine in Mainland France 2009–2010: Results of a National Vaccination Campaign. *Vaccine* 28 (51): 8157–8161.

Briggs, C., and M. Nichter. 2009. Biocommunicability and the Biopolitics of Pandemic Threats. *Medical Anthropology* 28 (3): 189–198.

Burges Watson, D., T. Moreira, and M. Murtagh. 2009. Little Bottles and the Promise of Probiotics. *Health* 13 (2): 219–234. https://doi.org/10.1177/1363459308099685.

Cohen, E. 2009. *A Body Worth Defending: Immunity, Biopolitics and the Apotheosis of the Modern Body.* Durham: Duke University Press.

Davis, M. 2017. 'Is It Going to be Real?' Narrative and Media on a Pandemic. *Forum Qualitative Sozialforschung/Forum: Qualitative Social Research* 18 (1). Online: http://nbn-resolving.de/urn:nbn:de:0114-fqs1701187.

Davis, M., and D. Lohm. Forthcoming. *Pandemics, Publics and Narrative.* New York: Oxford University Press.

Davis, M., P. Flowers, and N. Stephenson. 2013. 'We Had to Do What We Thought Was Right at the Time': Retrospective Discourse on the 2009 H1N1 Pandemic in the UK. *Sociology of Health & Illness* 36 (3): 369–382.

Davis, M., N. Stephenson, and P. Flowers. 2011. Compliant, Complacent or Panicked? Investigating the Problematisation of the Australian General Public in Pandemic Influenza Control. *Social Science & Medicine* 72 (6): 912–918.

Davis, M., P. Flowers, D. Lohm, E. Waller, and N. Stephenson. 2014. 'We Became Sceptics': Fear and Media Hype in General Public Narrative on the Advent of Pandemic Influenza. *Sociological Inquiry* 84 (3): 499–518.

Davis, M., P. Flowers, D. Lohm, E. Waller, and N. Stephenson. 2016. Immunity, Biopolitics and Pandemics: Public and Individual Responses to the Threat to Life. *Body & Society* 22 (4): 130–154.

Fineberg, H. 2008. Preparing for Avian Influenza: Lessons from the 'Swine Flu Affiar'. *The Journal of Infectious Diseases* 197 (1): S14–S18.

Galarce, E., S. Minsky, and K. Viswanath. 2011. Socioeconomic Status, Demographics, Beliefs and A(H1N1) Vaccine Uptake in the United States. *Vaccine* 29 (32): 5284–5289.

Giddens, A. 1998. Risk Society: The Context of British Politics. In *The Politics of Risk Society,* ed. J. Franklin. Cambridge: Polity.

Green, A. 2014. West Africa Struggles to Contain Ebola Outbreak. *The Lancet* 383, 5 April.

Hilton, S., and E. Smith. 2010. Public Views of the UK Media and Government Reaction to the 2009 Swine Flu Pandemic. *BMC Public Health* 10: 697.

Holland, K., and W. Blood. 2012. Public Responses and Reflexivity During the Swine Flu Pandemic in Australia. *Journalism Studies iFirst.* https://doi.org/10.1080/1461670X.2012.744552.

Joffe, H. 2011. Public Apprehension of Emerging Infectious Diseases: Are Changes Afoot? *Public Understanding of Science* 20 (4): 446–460.

Kiviniemi, M., P. Ram, L. Kozlowski, and K. Smith. 2011. Perceptions of and Willingness to Engage in Public Health Precautions to Prevent 2009 H1N1 Influenza Transmission. *BMC Public Health* 11 (1): 152. https://doi.org/10.1186/1471-2458-11-152.

Koteyko, N. 2009. 'I Am a Very Happy, Lucky Lady, and I Am Full of Vitality!' Analysis of Promotional Strategies on the Websites of Probiotic Yoghurt Producers. *Critical Discourse Studies* 6 (2): 111–125.

Lin, L., E. Savoia, F. Agboola, and K. Viswanath. 2014. What Have We Learned About Communication Inequalities During the H1N1 Pandemic: A Systematic Review of the Literature. *BMC Public Health* 14 (1): 484. https://doi.org/10.1186/1471-2458-14-484.

Martin, E. 1994. *Flexible Bodies: Tracking Immunity in American Culture from the Days of Polio to the Age of AIDS*. Boston: Beacon Press.

Martin, A. 2010. Microchimerism in the Mother(land): Blurring the Borders of Body and Nation. *Body & Society* 16 (3): 23–50.

Mitchell, T., D.L. Dee, C.R. Phares, et al. 2011. Non-Pharmaceutical Interventions During an Outbreak of 2009 Pandemic Influenza A (H1N1) Virus Infection at a Large Public University, April–May 2009. *Clinical Infectious Diseases* 52 (1): S138–S145.

National Health Service. 2009. Important Information About Swine Flu. Edited by Wales National Health Services for England, Scotland and Northern Ireland.

Nerlich, B., and N. Koteyko. 2008. Balancing Food Risks and Food Benefits: The Coverage of Probiotics in the UK National Press. *Sociological Research Online* 13 (3): 1.

Nerlich, B., and N. Koteyko. 2012. Crying Wolf? Biosecurity and Metacommunication in the Context of the 2009 Swine Flu Pandemic. *Health & Place* 18 (4): 710–717. https://doi.org/10.1016/j.healthplace.2011.02.008.

Presanis, A., R. Pebody, B. Paterson, B. Tom, P. Birrell, A. Charlett, and M. Lipsitch. 2011. Changes in Severity of 2009 Pandemic A/H1N1 Influenza in England: A Bayesian Evidence Synthesis. *BMJ* 343: d5408. https://doi.org/10.1136/bmj.d5408.

Robotham, Julie and Jonathan Pearlman. 2009. Global Alarm as Killer Swine Flu Spreads. *The Sydney Morning Herald*, 27 April. Online: http://www.smh.com.au/world/global-alarm-as-killer-swine-flu-spreads-20090426-ajjo.html.

Rose, N. 2007. *The Politics of Life Itself: Biomedicine, Power and Subjectivity in the Twenty-First Century*. Princeton: Princeton University Press.

Rubin, G., R. Amlot, L. Page, and S. Wessely. 2009. Public Perceptions, Anxiety, and Behaviour Change in Relation to the Swine Flu Outbreak: Cross Sectional Telephone Survey. *British Medical Journal* 339 (Online First).

Stephenson, N., M. Davis, P. Flowers, E. Waller, and C. MacGregor. 2014. Mobilising 'Vulnerability' in the Public Health Response to Pandemic Influenza. *Social Science and Medicine* 102: 10–17.

Ungar, S. 2003. Misplaced Metaphor: A Critical Analysis of the 'Knowledge Society'. *Canadian Review of Sociology* 40 (3): 331–347.

Ungar, Sheldon. 2008. Global Bird Flu Communication: Hot Crisis and Media Reassurance. *Science Communication* 29 (4): 472–497.

Van, D., M. McLaws, J. Crimmins, R. MacIntyre, and H. Seale. 2010. University Life and Pandemic Influenza: Attitudes and Intended Behaviour of Staff and Students towards Pandemic (H1N1) 2009. *BMC Public Health* 10 (1): 130. https://doi.org/10.1186/1471-2458-10-130.

Waller, E., M. Davis, and N. Stephenson. 2016. Australia's Pandemic Influenza 'Protect' Phase: Emerging Out of the Fog of Pandemic. *Critical Public Health* 26 (1): 99–113.

White, S., R. Petersen, and J. Quinlivan. 2010. Pandemic (H1N1) 2009 Influenza Vaccine Uptake in Pregnant Women Entering the 2010 Influenza Season in Western Australia. *MJA* 193: 405–407.

World Health Organization. 2009. WHO, 2009 World Now at the Start of 2009 Influenza Pandemic. Online: http://www.who.int/mediacentre/news/statements/2009/h1n1_pandemic_phase6_20090611/en/index.html.

World Health Organization. 2011. Implementation of the International Health Regulations (2005). Report of the Review Committee on the Functioning of the International Health Regulations (2005) in Relation to Pandemic (H1N1) 2009. Report by the Director-General. Geneva: World Health Organisation.

World Health Organization. 2014. Statement on the 1st Meeting of the IHR Emergency Committee on the 2014 Ebola Outbreak in West Africa. Online: http://www.who.int/mediacentre/news/statements/2014/ebola-20140808/en/.

World Health Organization. 2016. Fifth Meeting of the Emergency Committee Under the International Health Regulations (2005) Regarding Microcephaly, Other Neurological Disorders and Zika Virus. http://www.who.int/mediacentre/news/statements/2016/zika-fifth-ec/en/.

Yi, S., D. Nonaka, M. Nomoto, J. Kobayashi, and T. Mizue. 2011. Predictors of the Uptake of A (H1N1) Influenza Vaccine: Findings from a Population-Based Longitudinal Study in Tokyo. *PLoS ONE* 6 (4): e18893.

CHAPTER 4

Enacting Pandemics: How Health Authorities Use the Press—And *Vice Versa*

Kristian Bjørkdahl and Benedicte Carlsen

Abstract Pandemics and other public health crises typically attract a great deal of media attention, and some scholars have argued that they are prime examples of "media hypes." That was certainly true of the 2009 pandemic, which in several countries became the biggest news story of that year. But how are pandemics mediated, and why are they mediated in that way? In this chapter, we draw on interviews with public health officials and newspaper editors in Norway, to explore how these parties co-enacted the drama that was the 2009 pandemic. We find that many of the decisions taken by the health authorities were motivated by a particular set of assumptions about how the media works, but at the same time, that the media deny the accuracy of these assumptions.

Keywords COVID-19 · Media coverage · Health officials · Mediation · Pandemic communication

K. Bjørkdahl (✉) · B. Carlsen
Uni Research Rokkan Centre, Bergen, Norway
e-mail: kristian.bjorkdahl@sum.uio.no

B. Carlsen
e-mail: benedicte.carlsen@uib.no

© The Author(s) 2019
K. Bjørkdahl and B. Carlsen (eds.), *Pandemics, Publics, and Politics*,
https://doi.org/10.1007/978-981-13-2802-2_4

43

Almost invariably, pandemics and other public health crises become big news stories. We need only think of SARS, the foot-and-mouth epidemic, the tsunami disaster, the avian flu, the 2009 flu pandemic, the Ebola epidemic, or the Zika outbreak, to understand that such episodes tend to become so-called "media hypes"—periods of intense mediation that arise whenever an issue "develop[s] a life of its own, creating huge news waves on one specific topic" (Vasterman 2005: 508; see also Vasterman 2018).

The question of why some issues become big news stories, and what that in turn means, is by no means new. In fact, this chiasmus—what causes news, and what does news in turn cause—has been a recurring object of study in journalism and media studies, with *loci classici* such as Galtung and Ruge's (1965) study of "news factors/values," McCombs and Shaw's (1972) study of "agenda-setting," and Downs' (1972) study of "issue-attention cycles." In much of this research, however, there has been a certain tendency to speak of news as though it were a natural phenomenon. As Stuart Hall once remarked, we often "speak of 'the news' as if events select themselves," as if the question of "which 'news angles' are most salient [is] divinely inspired" (Hall, cited in O'Neill and Harcup 2009: 163). The events that end up as news represent, however, only a tiny proportion of a great multitude, and we can only properly understand how they end up as such if we highlight the actors, institutions, and processes that *make* news of this small number of issues.

In fairness, there have been attempts to assimilate this way of thinking with the idea of media hypes. Wien and Elmelund-Præstekær argue, for instance, that we cannot distinguish neatly between news *events* and news *making*: "Politicians and their spin doctors know how the media work," they argue, "and they utilize this knowledge in order to get as much publicity as they can" (2009: 185). While we believe this represents a step in the right direction, it still makes news making sound like an overly mechanistic affair: If politicians know how the media *work*, and they *utilize this knowledge in order to* get what they want, the media is seen—simplistically—as a mere instrument.

In this chapter, we start from the idea that our making news of pandemics and other public health crises can usefully be viewed as a sort of drama—in other words, that the mediation of such episodes resembles the enactment of a play, for which the media functions as a stage, or even in some ways an entire theater. We take this performance metaphor from Stephen Hilgartner (2000), who in turn finds inspiration in Erving Goffman (1959). For our purposes, to propose that the mediation of pandemics and other public health crises can be seen as a drama is not just to say that such crises tend to be communicated as riveting plots, dotted with heroes, victims, and villains, which confront us with vertiginous climaxes and reassuring resolutions—although that does indeed tend to be the case. It is, more importantly, to place into focus the various actors and institutions responsible for enacting this drama on the media stage.

To see such crises as dramas means to see them, at least in part, as conflicts—or at the very least, as dynamic and interest-driven interactions. No actor or institution can singlehandedly stage a public health crisis, just as a play proper cannot be staged by a single person. Rather, different actors and institutions, in their different capacities, and with varying levels of expertise—not to mention divergent interests and purposes—must interact. The stage actors might not obediently follow the director's lead, however, and the director might in turn be making a soup of the playwright's intentions. Meanwhile, owners and managers keep imposing restrictions on the production, while audiences and critics remain notoriously volatile.

This combination of characteristics—on the one hand, that public health crises tend to become media hypes, and on the other, that they are dramas saturated with diverging interests—create a particular set of challenges for those tasked with responding to pandemics and other public health crises, notably the health authorities. In a modern society, pandemic response is simply not possible without the media, and if such response is to be effective, the authorities rely on getting their message across. Communication failure overlaps with a failure of pandemic response. As Jonathan Quick suggests, "health communication lies at the heart of epidemic control" (2018: 22).

Not much is known, however, about *how* authorities attempt to use the media for their purposes during pandemics and other public health crises, nor to what extent politicians and their spin doctors *actually* "know how the media work." We will not be in a position to helpfully critique and correct crisis communication efforts until we understand the moves and motives of those who communicate—all those who stage the play, as it were. What is the objective of the health authorities in situations like these, and what means do they use? How, and to what extent, do the media accommodate those goals, and with what motivations?

With the aim of understanding how authorities and media co-produced the drama that was the 2009 pandemic—officially termed A(H1N1)pdm09—we present here an interview-based study of why health authorities and media editors in Norway acted as they did during the episode. Our study reveals that the health authorities made assumptions about the media that did not match the media's own idea of what they were doing. More concretely, the health authorities were motivated by the perceived importance of "grabbing the information space," in an effort to ward off other—"inferior"—sources and messages. Media editors, however, deny the logic of this assumption. We find, in other words, that the various actors involved in the co-production of this play had somewhat different conceptions of the production at hand, and we stipulate that this might have left the audience rather confused about what the play was really about (for more on the audience response, see Bjørkdahl and Carlsen 2018).

MINOR PANDEMIC, MAJOR RESPONSE

The mediation of the flu began on April 25, 2009, the day after the World Health Organization (WHO) had issued a worldwide Disease Outbreak Notice, declaring that a new influenza had been detected in Mexico. Epidemiologists expect flu pandemics to occur with a certain interval, and after the Avian flu outbreak of 2005 had not reached pandemic scales, public health officials were by 2009 anxiously anticipating the next one. When news arrived from Mexico, the WHO's response was thus swift and forceful. A "public health emergency of international concern" was declared, and the pandemic alert level was raised, first from 3 to 4, and then from 4 to 5, by April 29. On June 11, it was raised again, to Level 6, which meant that a pandemic was declared (CDC 2010). The WHO's lead was quickly followed up by the various national health authorities, who turned to their respective populations with information and advice—in general by way of the media. In Norway, from where we draw our material, the health authorities informed the public through press conferences, daily reports and press releases, participation in radio, press, and TV interviews and debates, op-eds in the newspapers, as well as their own website, *pandemi.no* (see Chapter 6 of this volume). With a few exceptions, communication about the pandemic in Norway resembled that in many other countries (see Carlsen and Glenton 2016).

On Monday 27 April, only a few days after news about the flu first broke, the Norwegian health authorities entered the scene with a major press conference featuring the main health authorities involved. Press conferences are rare events in Norwegian public health work, and this one was quite exceptional. It took place in a large venue in "Regjeringskvartalet," the government quarter, was live streamed, and contained somber presentations by the Minister of Health, the Health Director (i.e. the chief public health bureaucrat), and an epidemiological expert at the National Institute of Public Health. The representative of the Institute and the Health Director both emphasized the uncertain state of the knowledge about the disease, but the latter in addition informed the public of a "worst case" scenario which was embedded in Norway's official pandemic plan. This scenario estimated that 1.2 million Norwegians—roughly a quarter of the country's population at the time—could be contaminated by the disease and that as many as 13,000 Norwegians might die. Accompanying this message were images on a big screen of health workers in protective gear, who appeared to be placing a corpse in a coffin.

This set off a veritable flood of news coverage, which continued, in three main waves, throughout 2009. During the duration of the pandemic, the coverage spanned more or less all sorts of news genres, latching the flu onto a great variety of other stories—from the preparedness of hospitals, to the risk of contamination during a major football tournament, to new hand-cleaning practices in schools and kindergartens, and so on. The coverage as a whole did not leave out critical voices, and a great deal of the authorities' communication consisted in responding to complaints and criticisms. "The health authorities" denotes here Ministry of Health and Care Services, the Directorate of Health, an executive and regulatory agency charged with enacting public health policy, and the Norwegian Institute of Public Health, which is primarily a research institution, but which has increasingly taken on a mandate of research communication, recommendations, and science advice. Norway being a small country, these governmental agencies are very tight-knit, and had as their stated goal to speak with one voice during the pandemic. The news media landscape is rather more diverse, and consists of largely depoliticized party presses that span from tabloids, such as *Verdens Gang* and *Dagbladet* to more serious outlets like *Aftenposten* and *Dagens Næringsliv*, in addition to a great number of local newspapers and radio stations.

For the present study, we have interviewed 6 media editors and 12 representatives of the health authorities, the majority of interviews lasting approximately an hour. The selection of media was somewhat random, but did include both tabloid and reputable outlets, both nationally and regionally. The selection of health authorities is more complete, and includes interviews with the heads of the relevant agencies, their deputies, as well as communication officers and senior researchers. In the case of the editors, all but one were interviewed twice, at the beginning and towards the end of our project. The representatives of the health authorities were interviewed only once, but some were followed up via e-mail.

GRABBING THE "INFORMATION SPACE"—WITH *GRAVITAS*

In our interviews, it quickly transpired that the health authorities' communication efforts during the pandemic had sprung from a communications strategy that was widely shared among all the relevant agencies. In essence, the strategy rested on an assumption that the authorities should communicate *openly and at an early stage*, in order to "grab the information space," as several of our informants put it. The authorities believed that by "filling" the media with messages they considered desirable, they would "crowd out" other, less reliable, sources of information. In practice, this objective was combined with the decision to communicate very solemnly—one might even say gravely—about the disease. This consideration rested on the assumption that if they did not communicate with sufficient seriousness, they could face an even more somber scenario later, if the disease turned out to be serious. It was better to "push the big button," as the Ministry's secretary general said, even if that meant one had to "tone things down afterwards." She added, "I would rather face criticism for being too dramatic than for being too *un*dramatic" (A1). The Minister said almost precisely the same thing: "I would rather be criticized for exaggerating this, if it turned out *not* to be that bad, than be criticized for minimizing it if it *was* bad" (A2). The Director of Health likewise stated, "You can't risk the attitude that it probably isn't serious" (A5).

If this, by 2009, had become the general attitude among the health authorities, a research director at the Institute of Public Health explained that the imperative to communicate openly and at an early stage reflected quite recent changes in her institution's approach to public communication. "In the old days, our director did most [of our communication]," she said, and explained that they, just a few decades ago, had been far more reserved in their approach to the media. In the last 15 years or so, she explained, "we have grown aware that since everything gets out anyway, better that it should come from us than from some other party – and this probably describes our thinking in 2009" (A3).

The Institute's spokesperson emphasized the same point, noting that 20 years ago, "certain reports would be marked 'Not to be published except with the approval of...' Now, however, it is important to get as much information as we can out there, as fast as we can, quality-controlled as well as we can in the short time we have available." He said that this new "proactive relation to the media" represented a "*total* turnaround in this area," and added that, "When the pandemic came, this was the kind of thinking we had in our spines, that *we ought to tell them what we know*" (A4).

Occasionally, this communicative imperative was connected to civic ideals like transparency, knowledge-sharing, etc., but as a rule, our informants justified it strategically. To communicate openly and at an early stage would quite simply yield better results; it would put the authorities in a better position. "There is always someone who knows," the research director noted, "and [the media] can easily get a hold of someone with an opinion. Not to mention that news travels very fast" (A3). Then she added the phrase that recurred in most all of our interviews with the health authorities: "If we don't grab the information space there will always be someone else there to do it" (A3).

She motivated this by saying that the health authorities might, at a later stage, find themselves in a situation "where we are asked to explain and defend ourselves" and that would be a much easier task, she said, if they did not have to "try to change a picture that someone has already created" (A3). In other words, she emphasized the importance of the power of definition: Only by getting on the media stage early, with seriousness but without pretense, could *they* be the ones to define what this disease was all about. If the pandemic is seen as a drama, we have found an assumption that one needs to put one's own stamp on the production, quickly and firmly, before someone else comes along and does precisely that.

The Health Director rehearsed the same message in justifying the decision to organize the first press conference: "If you don't grab the information space, there will in any case be a lot of information out there, but *other* sources will be providing that information." He used a similar logic when justifying their practice of frequent press briefs. Had they not held these briefs, the media coverage would have been dominated by views with which the health authorities strongly disagreed, he said, and added that "the press briefs guarantee that we, who after all command a system that can actually understand the situation, are the media's most important informants" (A5).

The announcement of the infamous worst-case scenario was justified with reference to a similar rationale. Since that scenario could already be found in public documents, the director noted, a pre-emptive move was the only sensible one. "The media would no doubt get their hands on it – and this much we know, that if the media finds stuff like this, there will be a story" (A5). His words were echoed by his assistant director of communications, who said that, "if we hadn't informed the public what we had planned for, someone would have figured it out" (A6). The Ministry's secretary general made even more clear the dangers of not communicating *openly and at an early stage*: "Had we *not* done that, the next story would have been: 'Here is what the Ministry is hiding'" (A1).

The authorities assumed, in other words, that the media would be "digging for dirt"—that their first impulse would be to sniff out a scandal or instance of misconduct that would play well on the front page. This assumption appears to have taken a firm hold of our informants, which meant, among other things, that they reflexively converted their communications strategy into an evaluative statement after-the-fact. The secretary general referred, for instance, to "all those on the outside who wanted big stories on some special interest issues connected to the pandemic," and argued, as though she were describing what had actually happened, that, "Because we filled the space with what we had of professional knowledge, it was harder for them to get their messages across, and only those who really had a solid message really got across, or had an impact" (A1).

What would have happened had the authorities not chosen this strategy, we cannot know. But it is certainly the case that Norwegian media, at least after a while, came to be filled with all sorts of messages and "special interests." In fact, the media coverage of the pandemic allowed not just for the authorities' own "professional knowledge," but also for various criticisms, coming from actors in many different capacities, including doctors and professors of medical ethics and social medicine, all the way to outright conspiracy theories, which held that the disease and/or the vaccine was a conspiracy enacted by an unholy alliance between Big Pharma, the WHO, and our national health authorities.

Nevertheless, there is no doubt that the imperative described above was in fact what motivated the authorities' communication during the pandemic, that this imperative was felt across the various agencies involved in handling the pandemic; and that they all justified it primarily with reference to strategic concerns. In our efforts to find out why this imperative had come to form such a hard core in the authorities' communications strategy—to the extent, in fact, that none of our informants saw any reason to correct it after the experience from 2009—three main factors came to light:

The *first* has to do with a general change in how all of these institutions approached public communication, which might in turn have to do with an even more general change in society as such. As our informants explained, there was a sense that one ought now to communicate more, more often, more willingly, sooner, and more "openly," which is to say, more transparently than one had in the past. In part, this was seen simply as a given, as an imperative that had emerged in the course of the last few decades. A few informants related it to changes in the journalistic field. They suggested that news media over time had been growing increasingly short on resources, and that reporters consequently had to dig out more "scandals" at a lesser cost, a development some of our informants connected to a general increase in the "pace" of news. In short, news moves faster than it used to, therefore the authorities have to do so as well.

The *second* factor had to do with a small number of concrete episodes, where the most influential people in the Norwegian health authorities felt they had made insights about "how the media work," as Wien and Elmelund-Præstekær put it. One particularly notable episode was the 2004 tsunami disaster, which befell a notable number of Norwegian tourists vacationing in Thailand, and which was handled poorly by the Norwegian government. "We were blindsided by it," said the secretary general at the Ministry (A1). That entailed a shift towards establishing a more proactive attitude to preparedness, to make sure that plans (which had existed also in 2004), were "alive," and then, in an attempt to succeed with the first goal, to knit the different governmental entities in the health sector more tightly together, so that they would speak with one voice and act as one body when the time came. We understand this effort to be one important reason why most all our informants in the health authorities use literally the same language when speaking about the 2009 response.

Finally, a *third* factor was theory. According to the assistant communications director at the Directorate, "We have based our work on
a theoretician called Peter Sandman, and there is one staffer in particular who has driven forth this way of thinking in our department" (A6).
She emphasized that they did not "work strictly according to a theory,"
but then went on to explain how their communication strategy during
the pandemic was in fact in line with Sandman's theories: "What's special
about [Sandman] is that he is very clear that you should not hold back
on anything, and not try to hide anything, and that was the background
for our being very clear about what we have prepared for, what we have
planned, what kind of scenarios we envisioned, the best and the worst"
(A6). Whatever the precise relation between communication theory and
practice in these institutions, the fact that they were so explicitly aware
that "their" strategy had been elaborated and defended in an academic
context is likely to have consolidated their faith in it.

First We Forward Information, Then We Criticize the Source

If this sums up some of the assumptions of one central group of actors
involved in staging the 2009 pandemic, we turn now to another group
who were important in that production: the media. Although the
media editors' perspective was certainly not wholly different from what
we found among the representatives of the health authorities, they did
depart from the latter in some significant, and perhaps surprising, ways.

Our informants in the media said, very uniformly, that the main
reason why the pandemic became such a big story, both in quantita-
tive terms and in terms of the journalistic rhetoric, was the authorities'
"drum-banging," in particular the infamous first press conference. When
the authorities make a move like that, the editors explained, it would be
almost irresponsible for news media not to "go big." The concern to
convey "information" from the authorities, is one of several functions of
the media in a situation like this, they pointed out. Another is criticism,
which here meant to investigate the background for the advice given, find
sources that had another take on the situation than the one presented by
the authorities, and so on. The editors, however, point to certain practically inevitable conditions which impose a chronological order on these
functions—in short, the critical function can only be performed after a
while. The media themselves have no competence to make independent

assessments on issues such as pandemics, and they also typically lack access to other good sources in the initial phase. Indeed, the editors explain that it is equally necessary for them to lean on the authorities in the first phase as it is to lean on a wider set of sources in the following one.

"We see it as the role of the media generally to convey central and important warnings issued from the authorities to the public," said one editor, but added that "another concern is to examine the authorities' exercise of power, which entails looking into what grounds they have to offer the advice they give the population" (M4). While most all the editors we interviewed touched on both of these two purposes—information and critique—they all also emphasized that the most important one, chronologically speaking, was the former.

They had several explanations why this was so. The first of them was an obligation of their occupation, which meant that they had no real choice about what to do after the first press conference. "The swine flu is a good example of an issue where the authorities struck a solemn chord from the very start," said one, and explained that, "It was pretty obvious that we were going to make this a priority ... when heavy actors like these ... including the Minister of Health come on the scene so strongly" (M4). The first press conference was in fact highlighted by *all* the editors as a highly significant event: "The turning point for us was that big press conference, where we understood that the authorities are taking this very seriously, and we were taken by this kind of duty to inform the public and be serious about our coverage of the issue" (M2). Another said that, "What took hold at our paper was a strong obligation to inform the public." The same editor explained that reflex as a practical expression of a general value of journalism: "This is a very strong desire in a situation where the whole population is under threat that the issue is: How we can inform in a proper way" (M3). One editor elaborated this point, saying that the first press conference set off the information reflex of the media: "When the authorities sound a national epidemics alarm, and present the kinds of scenarios they did in this case, they bring a certain gravity to the situation; it is made into a national matter, and for that reason the alarm goes off in the media" (M1). As they explained, the media's reaction to the first press conference was a duty of information, an obligation to "inform in a proper way." Given the *gravitas* with which the authorities first announced this new flu, the media coverage that ensued was simply a case of the media taking the authorities' seriousness seriously.

At the same time, the editors are keen to point out that this kind of "forwarding" of information from the authorities is just one of their two main functions, and that these two typically follow a certain order. As one editor lamented, "ideally, we should be doing both [information and critique] at the same time, but what typically happens in practice—and this is my experience after 20 years in this game—is that we, in a first, acute phase tend to simply forward what is communicated" (M4). She acknowledged that this might be the case particularly in small news organizations like her own, but based on experience from other, larger news media, insisted that it was a general trend: *First*, one forwards the authorities' message, in "informational" form; *then*, one gets down to questioning and criticizing it. One editor referred to this equation as "a sort of built-in dramaturgy," and as "classical news journalism": "First, you write about it, then in the next phase, you place the authorities under close scrutiny" (M3).

This explanation was repeated, with only minor alterations, by all the rest of the editors we interviewed. Although they sometimes referred to this dynamic almost as a natural fact, what they meant was that it was a product of the incentives that are typically at play in the newsroom. Limited resources means one simply lacks the manpower to fulfill both functions at the same time, at least not from the start. This is particularly impossible, the editors pointed out, with technical issues like a pandemic, since only very few news organizations employ designated health journalists with the competence to raise critical questions from the start. As one editor pointed out, "Most newspaper don't possess the competence among their in-house staff to assess whether the information provided by experts about a disease like this is accurate or not. We don't even have a designated health journalist!" (M5). Another said that, "I don't have the medical knowledge to judge whether what is said is correct or not" (M4).

The typical consequence of this is, again, that the media—especially in the first phase of the coverage—have no choice but to rely heavily on the official sources, in this case, the health authorities. "It's not so easy to be critical in this phase," said one editor, "because we don't have sources besides the authorities themselves. Later, obviously, other sources enter the picture, and the critical stance becomes more important" (M3). One editor argued that this should give no cause for concern, as "the authorities are, generally, very good sources. I mean, they have the expertise, and they are *supposed* to have that expertise, and for that reason alone, they are an obvious source for us" (M5).

There is in other words both a push and a pull here, both a practical reason and a professional one: News media on the one hand *must* rely on official sources in this first phase, but they also feel an *obligation* to do so. When important societal actors like the health authorities get on the stage—as they literally did during the above-mentioned press conference—the media feel obligated by the norms of their profession to report. As one editor stated, "In retrospect one might suggest that we ought to have problematized the authorities' alarm, but this is not so obvious; should we, from day one, or two or three or four, when the authorities used this kind of weaponry, not have reacted with gravity?" (M1). The same informant added that, although the first phase of coverage of the flu was a story "on the authorities' terms," it would not be relevant to criticize the media for being a mere mouthpiece to the government. Rather, he argued, "when there is this type of alarm, it is our job to contribute to informing the public in a broad way" (M1).

But just as it is part of the professional ethics of journalists to report "broadly" and forward the authorities' information, another part is to bring critical perspectives: "It is your job to balance, to draw up appropriate dimensions and introduce other voices, and to ask critical questions" (M1). All the editors underlined, however, that this function came only later. This again was explained with reference both to a professional value and to the incentives of the newsroom: On the one hand, it is a central part of journalism to question the authorities, on the other, "it is in the nature of news," as one informant said, "that it is no longer news if you keep reporting the same thing" (M4). News journalism, she added, "keeps looking for new angles, whether it's an improvement or a deterioration of the issue you have presented, or whether new aspects come up that might be interesting" (M4). So while the critical function was partly motivated by the journalistic obligation to hold the authorities accountable, another motivation, again, was resources. As the same editor explained, "For a small newspaper like ours, a serialized story like this makes good sense. To grab hold of a small number of issues, that's a good method for us, first because it allows us to create a [narrative] in a violent storm of information, but also because we can create a sense of in-depth knowledge on particular issues" (M4). In other words, the function to dig for dirt and come up with criticism is—just as the function of information—not just one of journalistic ideals, but also one of journalistic finances.

Working Out How the Media Work

The most important finding from these interviews, we believe, is that the health authorities and the media made quite different assumptions about how pandemics and other public health crises are enacted on the media's stage. In an attempt to be the playwrights of this drama, the authorities put great emphasis on going to the media at an early stage and to communicate broadly and openly—not "holding back on" or "trying to hide" anything, just as their preferred theoretician prescribed. This priority reveals, however, that the authorities—*contra* the pronouncement of Wien and Elmelund-Præstekær—do *not* necessarily "know how the media work."

In fact, the authorities' notion that "grabbing the information space" was a prerequisite for getting their message across, appears quite simply to be wrong. As the editors explain, they do not have the resources to question the authorities in this first phase, and hence, there is not necessarily a need to rush things. In technical issues like a pandemic, the media is going to want to hear the authorities' story anyway. Despite their reputation for always sniffing out a scandal—for always wanting, as the Institute's research director said, "something, anything, that can create a headline" (A3)—the media consider it their professional duty to forward the authorities' information in grave situations like a pandemic. The media count the authorities to be not just the first, but also the best, source on the matters such as these, and this insight could, we imagine, cause the authorities to readjust their communication strategy. Instead of *communicate openly and at an early stage*, one could perhaps consider *communicate honestly and at the appropriate time?*

The other aspect of the authorities' assumption appears to be equally wrong: Their decision to communicate openly and from an early stage did little to "ward off" other sources. In fact, despite the demonstrably important and in many ways unprecedented first press conference, not to mention the authorities' frequent press briefs, the media after a while did move on to using a wider set of sources, many of which were critical of the official health apparatus. Also, the media themselves—via its columnists, editorials, editorial choices of angles, etc.—increasingly cast a more critical light on the authorities' pandemic response and communication. According to the editors, this had little to do with this pandemic's particular course, but was rather an almost inevitable effect of the incentives at play in the newsroom—a "sort of built-in dramaturgy," as one editor put it. News media cannot keep running the same story with the same angle over time, because if they did, they would no longer be conveyors of *news*. Given the concrete incentives of a newsroom, then, they must do one of three things: Write the authorities' angle, write someone else's angle, or find a new story altogether.

It is thus our conclusion that the authorities in this case relied on a communication strategy that, in some important ways, did not understand "how the media work." Had they more profoundly taken into account the incentives of the newsroom, the authorities could probably have prevented the overly dramatic first wave of coverage, which was almost certainly a direct effect of their press conference. They could consequently have averted the need to backtrack, which arguably created a certain confusion as to the severity of the disease (Bjørkdahl and Carlsen 2017). They could, quite simply, have managed to stage a drama that was closer to their own vision.

REFERENCES

Bjørkdahl, Kristian, and Benedicte Carlsen. 2017. Fear of the Fear of the Flu: Assumptions About Media Effects in the 2009 Pandemic. *Science Communication* 39 (3): 358–381.

Bjørkdahl, Kristian, and Benedicte Carlsen. 2018. Pandemic Rhetoric and Public Memory: What People (Don't) Remember from the 2009 Swine Flu. In *Rhetorical Audience Studies and Reception of Rhetoric: Exploring Audiences Empirically*, ed. Jens Kjeldsen, 261–284. London: Palgrave Macmillan.

Carlsen, Benedicte, and Claire Glenton. 2016. The Swine Flu Vaccine, Public Attitudes, and Researcher Interpretations: A Systematic Review of Qualitative Research. *BMC Health Services Research* 16: 203.

CDC (Centers for Disease Control and Prevention). 2010. The 2009 H1N1 Pandemic: Summary Highlights, April 2009–April 2010. https://www.cdc.gov/h1n1flu/cdcresponse.htm.

Downs, Anthony. 1972. Up and Down with Ecology: The Issue-Attention Cycle. *Public Interest* 28: 38–50.

Galtung, Johan, and Mari Holmboe Ruge. 1965. The Structure of Foreign News. The Presentation of the Congo, Cuba, and Cyprus Crises in Four Norwegian Newspapers. *Journal of Peace Research* 2 (1): 64–91.

Goffman, Erving. 1959. *The Presentation of Self in Everyday Life*. New York: Anchor Books.

Hall, Stuart. 1973. The Determinations of News Photographs. In *The Manufacture of News: Deviance, Social Problems and the Mass Media*, ed. Stanley Cohen and Jock Young, 226–243. London: Constable.

Hilgartner, Stephen. 2000. *Science on Stage: Expert Advice as Public Drama*. Stanford: Stanford University Press.

McCombs, Maxwell, and Donald Shaw. 1972. The Agenda-Setting Function of Mass Media. *The Public Opinion Quarterly* 36 (2): 176–187.

O'Neill, Deirdre, and Tony Harcup. 2009. News Values and Selectivity. In *The Handbook of Journalism Studies*, ed. Karin Wahl-Jorgensen and Thomas Hanitzsch, 161–174. New York: Routledge.

Quick, Jonathan. 2018. *The End of Epidemics: The Looming Threat to Humanity and How to Stop It*. New York: St. Martin's Press.

Vasterman, Peter. 2005. Media-Hype: Self-Reinforcing News Waves, Journalistic Standards and the Construction of Social Problems. *European Journal of Communication* 20 (4): 508–530.

Vasterman, Peter. 2018. Introduction. In *From Media Hype to Twitter Storm: News Explosions and Their Impact on Issues, Crises, and Public Opinion*, ed. Peter Vasterman, 17–38. Amsterdam: Amsterdam University Press.

Wien, Charlotte, and Christian Elmelund-Præstekær. 2009. An Anatomy of Media Hypes: Developing a Model for the Dynamics and Structure of Intense Media Coverage of Single Issues. *European Journal of Communication* 24 (2): 183–201.

CHAPTER 5

"Disease Knows No Borders": Pandemics and the Politics of Global Health Security

Antoine de Bengy Puyvallée and Sonja Kittelsen

Abstract Since the 1990s, the threat of pandemics has gained increased prominence on policy-makers' agendas due to the emergence and resurgence of infectious diseases and an increasingly interconnected world. Encapsulated by the phrase "disease knows no borders," this new risk environment has led to the rise of a new global health security regime, codified in the 2005 International Health Regulations. It is based on a paradigm of rapid detection and response to outbreak events, and on a norm of collective action. Drawing on examples from the 2014–2015 Ebola epidemic, we argue that pandemic preparedness is not just a technical matter, but also a political and normative one. We show that the global health security regime carries tensions that reflect asymmetries in actors' capacities to put forward their priorities.

A. de Bengy Puyvallée (✉)
Center for Development and the Environment,
University of Oslo, Oslo, Norway
e-mail: a.d.b.puyvallee@sum.uio.no

S. Kittelsen
Institute of Health and Society, University of Oslo, Oslo, Norway
e-mail: sonja.kittelsen@medisin.uio.no

© The Author(s) 2019
K. Bjørkdahl and B. Carlsen (eds.), *Pandemics, Publics, and Politics*,
https://doi.org/10.1007/978-981-13-2802-2_5

Keywords COVID-19 · Securitization · Global health security · IHR · Ebola · Pandemic politics

"Disease knows no borders" is a phrase used so frequently by academics, politicians, and public health professionals that it has become a truism. The expression captures a renewed sense of vulnerability to the microbial world that has arisen since the 1990s, due to the emergence and resurgence of infectious diseases in an increasingly interconnected world. The concern with the public health and security consequences of infectious diseases has led to the development of a new global health security regime.[1] This new regime is encapsulated in the revised International Health Regulations (IHR 2005)—the international legal instrument in place to prevent and control the cross-border spread of infectious disease—and constitutes a paradigm shift in global health governance (Davies et al. 2015; Fidler 2005). Under the IHR (2005) governments are accountable to both their publics *and* the global community in managing outbreak events and are obliged to develop a set of core public health capacities to be able to detect, assess and respond to infectious disease emergence. The Regulations institutionalize a norm of global collaboration when it comes to epidemic control, based on a logic of rapid detection and response to outbreaks events, and placed under the authority of the World Health Organization (WHO) (Davies and Youde 2016: 2).

This new global health security regime marks a shift in how we understand and deal with the microbial world at the international level. It challenges "the traditional distinctions between local-global, traditional-human security, and domestic-international health" (Davies et al. 2015: 16). However, in so doing, it has also revealed a number of tensions in international efforts to manage epidemic and pandemic events, tensions that were made particularly apparent during the global response to the Ebola epidemic in 2014–2015. These relate to the types of measures favored by the international community in preparing for and responding to pandemic threats, and countries' willingness to comply with the IHR (2005) when their national interest could be threatened.

In this chapter, we argue that pandemic preparedness and response is not just a technical matter, but also a political and normative one. Our contribution brings an international dimension to the analysis of public responses to health crises by exploring their global aspects. We argue that the risk highlighted by the phrase "disease knows no borders" is the result of a social construction elaborated through a "power game" between actors with varying capacities of influence (Beck 2006: 333). We begin by tracing the emergence of the contemporary global health security regime by placing it in historical context and examining how a changing risk environment, summarized by the phrase "disease knows no borders," came to inform current international efforts to manage the microbial world. We then draw on examples from the Ebola epidemic of 2014–2015 to illustrate some of the tensions inherent in this new global health security regime, particularly the resistance of national interest, the privileging of containment over prevention policy, and of short-term, technology-based responses over longer-term engagements in strengthening health systems.

The Emergence of the Contemporary Global Health Security Regime

While the phrase "disease knows no borders" is often evoked to speak to a distinct contemporary vulnerability to the microbial world, the threat posed by infectious diseases is not new, nor are international efforts to control disease spread. International cooperation on countering the cross-border spread of infectious disease began in the second half of the nineteenth century (Harrison 2006). Responding to the unprecedented growth of international trade triggered by colonial expansion, European leaders sought to reduce trade barriers, including quarantine, while preventing what was seen as a new vulnerability—the international spread of infectious diseases. To tackle these issues, European nations got together in a series of international sanitary conventions. These conventions led to the emergence of an international health security regime, institutionalized with the creation of the WHO in 1948 and codified with the adoption of the International Sanitary Regulations in 1951, which were renamed the International Health Regulations in 1969. This "classical regime" (Fidler 2005: 327) required states to notify each other of the presence of a number of specific diseases in their territories, and to implement standardized and appropriate measures to control disease entry at their borders. Cooperation thus rested on the goodwill of states to share information and implement preventive measures that did not excessively disrupt international travel and trade.

By the 1990s, however, the IHR (1969) were no longer fit for purpose. A changing risk environment meant that the three diseases then covered by the Regulations—cholera, plague and yellow fever—no longer reflected the nature of the risks posed by infectious diseases in most countries. The discovery of new viruses, such as Ebola in 1976 and HIV in 1983, and the resurgence of old viruses in more volatile forms reinvigorated concerns over the threat posed by infectious diseases and underscored the inadequacy of international arrangements in place to manage them. Three elements supported a shift in the conceptualization of microbial threat (McInnes 2016): (1) there are new risks, including emerging diseases, against which science and innovation alone cannot protect us; (2) globalization connects the world in unprecedented ways and facilitates the spread of viruses, reducing the significance of political borders in containing pathogens; and (3) it is possible, through global cooperation, to limit these risks by setting up global surveillance mechanisms and rapid biomedical response capacities. While elements of this argument echo those advanced in the nineteenth century under the classical regime of international disease cooperation, what distinguishes contemporary concerns from those of the past is the increased frequency with which new diseases are being identified and the increased speed with which they can spread. The result has been a shift in how we understand and deal with the microbial world at the international level, a shift often summarized by the phrase "disease knows no borders."

The US Institute of Medicine's 1992 report, *Emerging Infections: Microbial Threats to Health in the United States* (Lederberg et al. 1992), played an instrumental role in advancing this new perspective. The report introduced the concept of emerging and re-emerging infectious diseases as a new public health and security threat to the United States. It argued that an infectious disease threat anywhere posed a potential threat everywhere due to a combination of natural and human-made factors that have increased the emergence and facilitated the spread of disease. Key to countering this threat was the ability to detect disease emergence early through the establishment of effective disease surveillance systems at both national and global levels.

The argument advanced in the 1992 Institute of Medicine report drew considerable political, public and media attention in the US and internationally, particularly when connected to a highly lethal virus that caused a horrific death: Ebola (King 2002: 769). Indeed, Andrew Lakoff (2017: 149) has described how the Ebola virus served "as a paradigm for the global threat posed by 'emerging viruses'" during this time period. The discovery of the virus in then-Zaire in 1976, recurring outbreaks in Africa, and an outbreak of Ebola amongst imported monkeys in Virginia in 1989 were central to the establishment and diffusion of this new perception of microbial threat. Recurring outbreaks of known infectious diseases and the emergence of new ones in the years that have followed, such as SARS in 2003 and the H5N1 avian influenza virus in 2005, have given further credibility to the threat of emerging and re-emerging infectious diseases (Davies et al. 2015). The risk posed by pandemic influenza has been particularly emblematic in this regard. The continuous circulation of the virus and the possibility of it mutating to inflict significant economic, political and societal disruption, have led to considerable attention paid to pandemic preparedness planning nationally and internationally. The past couple of decades have thus seen the rise of health on foreign and security policy agendas and new cooperative arrangements to manage the threat of infectious disease.

A New Global Health Security Regime

If we live in a borderless world subject to emerging threats, then global cooperation is required to ensure collective health security. The proclamation that "disease knows no borders" is thus not a politically neutral statement. It is both a reaction to a changed risk environment, and the embodiment of a particular understanding of these new risks and what measures are required to address them. It advocates for a global regime relying on shared responsibilities and on an approach to epidemic preparedness and control based on a combination of surveillance, control measures, and biomedical response (Davies and Youde 2016; Kamradt-Scott 2015). The IHR (2005) is the translation on the global scene of these political recommendations and reflects the growing understanding of infectious diseases as both a public health and security threat. Under the revised IHR, governments are accountable not only to their publics, but also to the global community. States are expected to develop a set of core public health capacities focused on detecting and containing outbreaks at source (Fidler 2005). In addition, the revised Regulations strengthen the WHO by enabling it to draw on both official and unofficial sources of information in the evaluation of a potential disease threat. If the situation is found to meet the relevant criteria, the WHO can independently declare a Public Health Emergency of International Concern and issue guidelines for control measures and response (Kamradt-Scott 2015). The new global health security regime thus allows the WHO to bypass—to a certain extent—*political borders* when it comes to global surveillance so that *information borders* do not prevent the detection of epidemics. The IHR (2005) also prohibit national authorities from taking unilateral measures in the event of a Public Health Emergency of International Concern that go against the advice of the WHO and that unnecessarily damage travel and trade. Finally, in the eventuality of a state failing to fulfill its obligations under the IHR, the IHR (2005) open the door for a collective response, enabling interventions by different global actors (the WHO and other UN agencies, states, non-governmental organizations and philanthropic foundations, for example) such as the set-up of pharmaceutical responses and biomedical countermeasures (Elbe 2014).

The revised IHR thus constitute a response to a changed risk environment, and mark a shift in international understandings of the threat posed by infectious diseases and the measures required at both national and international levels to mitigate it. They introduce a set of norms and obligations on states and the global community in addressing pandemic risk. Yet, this new global health security regime is also the result of a "power game" between actors with varying capacities of influence (Beck 2006: 333). It creates tensions when it comes to the understanding of security (state versus individual), the prioritization of policies in addressing microbial threat (rapid detection and containment versus prevention through a focus on the socio-economic aspects of infectious diseases), and the division of responsibilities in preventing, preparing for, and responding to epidemic events (domestic versus international). As we will show in the following section, these tensions were made explicit during the Ebola crisis.

Ebola and the Limits of Global Health Security

The Ebola epidemic in West Africa in 2014–2015 revealed the limits of contemporary arrangements to manage the cross-border spread of infectious disease. The delayed global response to the epidemic and the lack of in-country capacity to effectively curtail the spread of the virus led to much debate following the crisis as to why the epidemic occurred and who was responsible for it. We focus here on three issues that emerged during the Ebola crisis that illustrate the limitations of the current global health security regime: (1) the tension between national interest and collective action in managing pandemic threat; (2) the power relations at play in defining international priorities for global health security; and (3) the significance of security- and technology-based approaches in shaping epidemic and pandemic response.

Managing Outbreaks: Tensions Between National Interest and Collective Action

The tension between national interest and collective action in managing epidemic and pandemic threats has been an ongoing challenge in the current regime of global preparedness and is made particularly apparent in the relationship between the WHO and its member states. The WHO received colossal criticism for its management of the Ebola epidemic, particularly for its delayed declaration of a Public Health Emergency of International Concern. The epidemic appeared out of control by the time of the declaration and the number of registered cases had already far exceeded those of previous outbreaks. The WHO was primarily criticized for its unwillingness to challenge the information provided by impacted countries' health authorities and for its inability to act as an independent agency, as the IHR (2005) theoretically intended (Kamradt-Scott 2016). Several independent commissions mandated to review the Ebola crisis found the WHO dysfunctional and recommended urgent reforms to remedy this (see, for instance, the review from Gostin et al. 2016).

Yet, while WHO officials themselves acknowledged mistakes in the management of the epidemic, the WHO's response cannot be seen in isolation from its relationship to its member states. As Adam Kamradt-Scott (2016: 409) has noted, the organization has historically faced battles with its member states in maintaining its institutional autonomy to manage cross-border health threats. This was evidenced during the renegotiation of the IHR, when a number of states, including Canada, Norway, Russia, Switzerland, Samoa and the United States, expressed reservations about the independence exercised by the WHO in intervening in the 2003 SARS epidemic. Member states ultimately decided to reject draft proposals that would grant the WHO the equivalent autonomy in managing other public health emergencies in order to safeguard their sovereignty (Kamradt-Scott 2015: 134–135, 2016: 409).

During the 2009 H1N1 influenza pandemic, moreover, a number of states took unilateral control measures, such as bans on pork imports and massive pork culls, against the recommendations of the WHO and often without justification. The WHO also faced criticism for declaring the pandemic a Public Health Emergency of International Concern. The organization was accused of having overreacted to and exaggerated the H1N1 threat, and faced speculation as to whether it had based its decision-making on politics or commercial interests (see, for example, Council of Europe Parliamentary Assembly 2010).

This historical relationship between the WHO and its member states has contributed to an institutional culture at the WHO that has tended to adopt a careful attitude when it comes to questioning member states' sovereign decisions and is reflected in the WHO's Ebola response (Kamradt-Scott 2016). West African authorities initially toned down the outbreak's magnitude when they notified the WHO of the epidemic. Despite signs suggesting a direr situation, however, the WHO did not challenge these initial reports. Rather, and perhaps with the legacy of H1N1 in mind, WHO officials reportedly delayed invoking the IHR for fear of taking measures that could be interpreted as "hostile" (Kamradt-Scott 2016: 407). Similar to H1N1, moreover, several countries unilaterally implemented travel bans and travel restrictions despite the multiple recommendations from the WHO not to do so (WHO 2014). A study found that 23% of WHO member states prohibited foreigners who were recently in a country experiencing widespread Ebola transmission to enter their territories, and an additional 8% imposed other substantial travel restrictions (Rhymer and Speare 2016). Tensions between national interest and collective action are thus a recurring problem in the current global health security regime and a crucial factor explaining why the lessons drawn after the H1N1 pandemic are strikingly similar to those drawn after the Ebola outbreak (Ottersen et al. 2016).

Priority-Setting and Power Relations in Global Health Security

The Ebola crisis also revealed the weaknesses of affected countries' health systems and indeed, their neglect. This neglect is in part a consequence of the lack of international priority given to strengthening low- and middle-income countries' capacities to manage outbreak events, and a reflection of a global health security regime that has privileged disease containment and control measures over those of prevention (Rushton 2011).

As previously mentioned, under the IHR (2005), countries are expected to establish core capacities to be able to detect, assess and report outbreak events within their territories. States were initially given until 2012 to implement these measures, the deadline being subsequently extended to 2014. Yet, when the Ebola outbreak started in 2014, only 64 out of 196 states signatory to the IHR had reported that they had met the requirements. Guinea, Liberia, and Sierra Leone were amongst those countries that had not. Despite accusations of a lack of political will, it seems more likely that these countries simply did not have the resources to invest in the IHR (Davies et al. 2015: 128).

Low- and middle-income countries were promised financial and technical support to reinforce their health systems during the IHR revision process, and after the H1N1 pandemic, one of the main lessons learned was the need to strengthen IHR core public health capacities (Ottersen et al. 2016). However, donor bodies prioritized instead disease-specific programs, with little effect on strengthening these core capacities (Davies et al. 2015: 126). One such program was the polio eradication program which was by far the WHO's largest funded project in 2014, drawing up to 38% of the organization's staff in Africa (Fortner and Park 2017). In addition, the limited financial transfers that were directly aimed at developing IHR core capacities were themselves often narrowly focused, "addressing particular core capacities (e.g., early warning surveillance) as opposed to others (e.g., laboratory diagnostics and risk communication)" (Davies et al. 2015: 132).

As Simon Rushton (2011: 784–785) has noted, moreover, the IHR (2005) are built on a logic of disease containment and control, privileging the set-up of surveillance and emergency response capacities. While these activities are dependent on the capabilities of domestic health systems, they have tended to be "treated separately from the type of public health provision (which includes everything from the provision of potable water to public health education) that plays a vital role in the prevention of outbreaks" (Rushton 2011: 785). The result has been a "decoupling" of *containment measures* (for instance, detection mechanisms and rapid response capacity) from those of *prevention*. The predominant paradigm for global health security has thus been a state-centric one, higher-income countries securing their interests and ensuring their health security by containing diseases at their source, while limiting investments in issues prioritized by lower- and middle-income countries such as general health system strengthening to both prevent epidemics and address diseases *already* having a terrible impact on their populations' health (Davies 2008; Rushton 2011). The result of this power asymmetry has been a global health security regime essentially *reactive* to epidemics, raising pressing questions with respect to financing and responsibility sharing for global health security going forward.

Security- and Technology-Driven Response

The culmination of the slow national and international recognition of the Ebola epidemic and the lack of in-country capacities to effectively manage the outbreak led to an international response to the epidemic that was both security-focused and technology-driven. The Ebola outbreak became a crisis in the summer of 2014 when three things occurred: (1) the virus spread outside its epicenter with the repatriation of sick health workers; (2) the WHO declared the outbreak a Public Health Emergency of International Concern, recognizing the virus as a risk to states internationally; and (3) early containment strategies having failed, the international community began to mobilize response efforts in order to cope with the threat. This context facilitated the securitization of the Ebola crisis, i.e. its framing as a national and international security threat. Thus, on 18 September 2014, the United Nations Security Council declared the outbreak "a threat to international peace and stability" (UNSC 2014). Ebola's securitization created a sense of gravity and urgency, reinforcing a logic of short-term containment already privileged in the global health security regime:

> The process of securitization promotes the perception of an immediate, potentially irreversible danger that creates a perceived need for rapid response. In a situation perceived as an emergency, alternative policy options, such as long-term engagement with complex socioeconomic issues and political negotiations, for instance, appear less suitable. Demand increases for a quick fix to avert the imminent danger. (Roemer-Mahler and Elbe 2016: 492)

The securitization of the Ebola crisis had at least three concrete effects on the global response. First, it was instrumental in mobilizing exceptional resources to contain the virus. Altogether, the global response raised US$ 4.3 billion, an amount corresponding to the budget needed to lead prevention policies by building universal health services and maintaining them for three years in Guinea, Sierra Leone, and Liberia (Save the Children 2015: IV). Second, the securitization of Ebola allowed countries to bypass traditional protocols for humanitarian crisis management by involving the military. The United States, for instance, deployed 3000 soldiers to Liberia with the mission to implement the response directly (White House 2014), whilst other countries, such as the United Kingdom, relied on the military's extensive capacities to support their response's logistics (DFID 2014). Third, the securitization of an issue reinforces an "emergency modality of action" (Collier and Lakoff 2008: 17), privileging short-term solutions, donor-led and technology-based. Technological solutions include medical counter-measures such as experimental drugs and vaccines—a trend that Stefan Elbe has called the *pharmaceuticalization* of global health (Elbe 2010; Roemer-Mahler and Elbe 2016). They include also what Peter Redfield has coined the "standardized humanitarian tool-kit" (such as base camps and field hospitals), comprising emergency resources that can be deployed everywhere, independently of the local context (Redfield 2008: 160–161).

Often portrayed as politically neutral, cost-effective and the most efficient way to deal with a humanitarian crisis—including an epidemic— (Roemer-Mahler and Elbe 2016: 493), these technological resources showed, however, clear limitations during the Ebola crisis because of their incapacity to engage with social context and the resistance they provoked. The WHO estimated, for instance, that between 60 and 80% of the infections during the Ebola outbreak were due to funeral rituals and the washing of dead bodies, these practices constituting one of the "factors that contributed to undetected spread of the Ebola virus and impeded rapid containment" (WHO 2015). Yet, because of its technological focus, the international response included few education and risk-reduction programs aimed at understanding these practices and proposing alternative solutions adapted to the local cultural context (Manguvo and Mafuvadze 2015; Richards 2016). In coordinating the global response in Sierra Leone, the UK, for instance, dedicated only 3% of its budget to do so (DFID 2014). Consequently, the technological solutions available were often not appropriate to the local context because, as recalled by the WHO, "when technical intervention cross purposes with entrenched cultural practices, culture always wins" (WHO 2015).

This securitized response to the Ebola epidemic is in many respects a logical outcome of the current global health security regime that has privileged national interest over collective action, containment over prevention, and short-term, technology-based responses over longer-term engagements in strengthening health systems. Indeed, while the revised IHR have introduced a new set of norms and obligations on the international community in mitigating pandemic risk, as this section has demonstrated, state interest and donor priorities have been influential in shaping the management of pandemic preparedness at international level. The result has been a regime underpinned by a security logic, essentially reactive to outbreak events, and in many respects disconnected from local context.

CONCLUSION

The international community's engagement with the microbial world has changed significantly since the turn of the century. The continued emergence and spread of known and novel viruses, facilitated by processes of globalization, has led to a shift in how states collectively negotiate the threat of infectious disease spread. This shift has been exemplified by the revision of the IHR—the key international legal instrument underpinning the contemporary global health security regime.

The IHR (2005) represent a paradigm shift in global health governance, introducing a set of norms and responsibilities on states in providing for collective health security. Yet, while the revised IHR and the changed risk environment in which they respond to challenge the significance of political borders in managing epidemics, as the Ebola outbreak in West Africa illustrated, in many respects, these borders continue to hold significance. Sovereignty and national interest continue to hold powerful sway in collective pandemic preparedness and response efforts, made no more apparent than in the relationship between the WHO and its member states in responding to the Ebola outbreak. The security logic underpinning the contemporary global health security regime, moreover, has led to a favoring of reactionary approaches to infectious disease emergence rather than preventive ones. The consequence has been a favoring of short-term, technical fixes over longer-term, more integrated engagements in building up countries' capacities to effectively mitigate outbreak events, and a predominant approach to pandemic preparedness through the lens of securitization.

NOTE

1. Steven Krasner (1982: 186) has defined the term regime as "sets of implicit or explicit principles, norms, rules and decision making procedures around which actors' expectations converge."

REFERENCES

Beck, Ulrich. 2006. Living in the World Risk Society. *Economy and Society* 35 (3): 329–345.

Collier, Stephen J., and Andrew Lakoff. 2008. The Problem of Securing Health. In *Biosecurity Interventions*, ed. Andrew Lakoff and Stephen Collier, 7–32. New York: Columbia University Press.

Council of Europe Parliamentary Assembly. 2010. The Handling of the H1N1 Pandemic: More Transparency Needed. *AS/Soc* (2010) 12, 23 March.

Davies, Sara E. 2008. Securitizing Infectious Disease. *International Affairs* 84 (2): 295–313.

Davies, Sara E., Adam Kamradt-Scott, and Simon Rushton. 2015. *Disease Diplomacy: International Norms and Global Health Security*. Baltimore: Johns Hopkins University Press.

Davies, Sara E., and Jeremy Youde (eds.). 2016. *The Politics of Surveillance and Response to Disease Outbreaks: The New Frontier for States and Non-State Actors*. London: Routledge.

DFID. 2014. UK Response to the Ebola Crisis in Sierra Leone and the Region. https://goo.gl/iSjx7x.

Elbe, Stefan. 2010. *Security and Global Health*. Lonon: Polity.

Elbe, Stefan. 2014. The Pharmaceuticalisation of Security: Molecular Biomedicine, Antiviral Stockpiles, and Global Health Security. *Review of International Studies* 40 (5): 919–938.

Fidler, David P. 2005. From International Sanitary Conventions to Global Health Security: The New International Health Regulations. *Chinese Journal of International Law* 4 (2): 325–392.

Fortner, Robert, and Alex Park. 2017. Bill Gates Won't Save You from the Next Ebola. *Huffington Post*, 30 April. http://www.huffingtonpost.com/entry/ebola-gates-foundation-public-health_us_5900a8c5e4b0026db1dd15e6?n-cid=engmodushpmg00000004.

Gostin, Lawrence O., Oyewale Tomori, Suwit Wibulpolprasert, Ashish K. Jha, Julio Frenk, Suerie Moon, Joy Phumaphi, Peter Piot, Barbara Stocking, Victor J. Dzau, and Gabriel M. Leung. 2016. Toward a Common Secure Future: Four Global Commissions in the Wake of Ebola. *PLoS Medicine* 13 (5): 1–15.

Harrison, Mark. 2006. Disease, Diplomacy and International Commerce: The Origins of International Sanitary Regulation in the Nineteenth Century. *Journal of Global History* 1 (2): 197.

Kamradt-Scott, Adam. 2015. *Managing Global Health Security: The World Health Organization and Disease Outbreak Control*. London: Palgrave Macmillan.

Kamradt-Scott, Adam. 2016. WHO's to Blame? The World Health Organization and the 2014 Ebola outbreak in West Africa. *Third World Quarterly* 37 (3): 401–418.

King, Nicholas B. 2002. Security, Disease, Commerce: Ideologies of Postcolonial Global Health. *Social Studies of Science* 32 (5/6): 763–789.

Krasner, Stephen D. 1982. Structural Causes and Regime Consequences: Regimes as Intervening Variables. *International Organization* 36 (2): 185–205.

Lakoff, Andrew. 2017. *Unprepared: Global Health in a Time of Emergency*. Berkeley: University of California Press.

Lederberg, Joshua, Robert E. Shope, and Stanley C. Oaks. 1992. *Emerging Infections: Microbial Threat to Health in the United States*. US Institute of Medicine.

Manguvo, Angellar, and Benford Mafuvadze. 2015. The Impact of Traditional and Religious Practices on the Spread of Ebola in West Africa: Time for a Strategic Shift. *The Pan African Medical Journal* 22 (1): 9.

McInnes, Colin. 2016. Crisis! What Crisis? Global Gealth and the 2014–15 West African Ebola Outbreak. *Third World Quarterly* 37 (3): 380–400.

Ottersen, Trygve, Steven J. Hoffman, and Gaëlle Groux. 2016. Ebola Again Shows the International Health Regulations Are Broken. *American Journal of Law & Medicine* 42 (2–3): 356–392.

Redfield, Peter. 2008. Vital Mobility and the Humanitarian Kit. In *Biosecurity Interventions*, ed. Andrew Lakoff and Stephen Collier, 147–172. New York: Columbia University Press.

Rhymer, Wendy, and Rick Speare. 2016. Countries' Response to WHO's Travel Recommendations during the 2013–2016 Ebola Outbreak. *Bulletin of the World Health Organization* 95 (1): 10–17.

Richards, Paul. 2016. *Ebola: How a People's Science Helped End an Epidemic*. London: Zed Books.

Roemer-Mahler, Anne, and Stefan Elbe. 2016. The Race for Ebola Drugs: Pharmaceuticals, Security and Global Health Governance. *Third World Quarterly* 37 (3): 487–506.

Rushton, Simon. 2011. Global Health Security: Security for Whom? Security from What? *Political Studies* 59 (4): 779–796.

Save the Children, UK. 2015. A Wake Up Call. Lessons from Ebola for the World's Health Systems.

UNSC. 2014. Resolution 2177, Adopted by the Security Council at Its 7268th Meeting, on 18 September 2014.

White House. 2014. Fact Sheet: U.S. Response to the Ebola Epidemic in West Africa. The White House, Office of the Press Secretary, 16 September. https://obamawhitehouse.archives.gov/the-press-office/2014/09/16/fact-sheet-us-response-ebola-epidemic-west-africa.

WHO. 2014. Statement from the Travel and Transport Task Force on Ebola Virus Disease Outbreak in West Africa. http://www.who.int/mediacentre/news/statements/2014/ebola-travel/en/.

WHO. 2015. Factors that Contributed to Undetected Spread of the Ebola Virus and Impeded Rapid Containment.

CHAPTER 6

When Authority Goes Viral: Digital Communication and Health Expertise on *pandemi.no*

Kristian Bjørkdahl and Tone Druglitrø

Abstract One of the most pressing questions concerning pandemic preparedness and response today is how digital media can and will change pandemic communication: In a future pandemic, effective use of digital media could mean the difference between marginal and massive loss of human lives. In this chapter, we are interested in how medical experts can retain their status in an environment where many—partly because of digital media—have come to distrust mainstream expertise. We study the Norwegian health authorities' emergency web page, *pandemi.no*, and argue that it failed to use the affordances of the medium to develop features that acknowledge the actual concerns and voices of the public.

K. Bjørkdahl (✉)
Uni Research Rokkan Centre, Bergen, Norway
e-mail: kristian.bjorkdahl@sum.uio.no

T. Druglitrø
TIK Centre for Technology, Innovation and Culture,
University of Oslo, Oslo, Norway
e-mail: tone.druglitro@tik.uio.no

© The Author(s) 2019
K. Bjørkdahl and B. Carlsen (eds.), *Pandemics, Publics, and Politics*,
https://doi.org/10.1007/978-981-13-2802-2_6

Instead, it relied on a particular, fictional member of the public, which kept the website within a traditional—outdated—paradigm of public health communication.

Keywords COVID-19 · Digital communication · pandemi.no · Medical expertise · Media affordances

One of the most pressing questions concerning pandemic preparedness and response today is how digital media can and will change pandemic communication (Dosemagen and Aase 2016; Xiang et al. 2017). While our knowledge in this area remains sketchy (Wilson and Jumbert 2018), the stakes could hardly be higher: In a future pandemic, effective use of digital media could mean the difference between marginal and massive loss of human lives. Even though the full consequences of these media are not yet apparent, we cannot postpone the effort to think through what difference they might make for pandemic communication.

In traditional public health communication, the ideal message was one that caused a sufficient number of the public to take appropriate action, reducing as far as possible the loss of human lives. To this end, the health authorities took dissemination of "correct knowledge" to be a crucial aim of any sound containment strategy (Wagner-Egger et al. 2011: 462), and they saw themselves as the keepers of this knowledge. Their typical media of choice were posters, brochures, propaganda films, and—not least—the mass media (Angeli 2012: 203). In message as in medium, traditional public health communication assumed that the relation between experts and non-experts was decidedly *asymmetrical* and one-way. To simplify, with Collins and Evans, "it was inconceivable that decision-making in matters that involved science and technology could travel in any other direction than from the top down" (2002: 239).

With the coming of the World Wide Web, this paradigm of public health communication—which had already been under pressure for some time—appeared to be definitively overtaken by a successor paradigm that promised a more dialogical mode, one that would further ideals of "democratization of science" and "co-production of knowledge" (see Jasanoff 2004). As Gesser-Edelburg and Shir-Raz (2017) note in a recent book, there is today an increasing skepticism of scientific expertise, and digital media have played a central role in furthering this tendency. Digital media, they argue, presents an opportunity for "anyone" to share knowledge and communicate with practically any other, thereby generating a "wisdom of the crowd" (2017: 2). Whether or not *wisdom* is really the right word for the content that digital media generate (see e.g., Reagle 2015; Shanahan 2018), most now assume that these media are somehow caught up in—if not to say one central cause of—a shift toward greater symmetry between experts and non-experts.

This new situation presents pandemic communication with a conundrum, however, which Collins and Evans (2002) dub the "the expertise problem." In short, this refers to the issue of how science-based advice can—and whether it should—stand out from the supposed wisdom of the crowd. Gesser-Edelburg and Shir-Raz formulate the problem clearly: "[I]n a digital world where the public's voice is growing increasingly strong, how can health experts best exert influence to contain the global spread of infectious diseases?" (2017: xx). A central question for pandemic response today is thus how experts can retain their status as such in a media environment that works toward leveling the relation between experts and non-experts. To put it differently: How, in this new environment, can authorities still be seen as authoritative?

In this chapter, we start from the assumption that pandemic response only works if it rests on relevant expertise, but also that expertise only works if the health authorities can establish their authority vis-à-vis the public. In our view, this rhetorical task—which is traditionally conceived of as the *ethos* function of rhetorical discourse (see Prelli 1989)—always takes place within a particular social and cultural context. For example, it must be performed differently in a situation where many have come to question expertise than in one where experts are generally revered. Further, the function of establishing authority must necessarily take place with or through or from within the materiality of a particular medium, whether one's own voice in an open-air theatre, a printed book, the television, or a social media app. If we want to understand how certain actors come to be seen as credible, we cannot separate the acts of invention, arrangement and style (the three first "canons of rhetoric") from the particular medium that records and circulates our rhetorical creations. These two aspects—form and content—are necessary and intertwined elements of any act of communication.

In this chapter, we apply this way of seeing to *pandemi.no*, the Norwegian pandemic emergency web page, which went live during the 2009 pandemic. Focusing on how the specific technical features of the website combined with the rhetorical labor performed by the health authorities—that is, on how the health authorities took advantage of the so-called "affordances" (Hutchby 2001) of this particular medium—we will argue that *pandemi.no* demonstrably failed to develop features that acknowledge public voices. Instead of allowing the actual voices of the public to be seen and heard, the website made a stylized version of a fictional member of the public, which appeared most prominently as an implicit poser of questions in a Q&A section, but also more generally, as model reader of the site (Eco 1979). This meant the website remained firmly within a traditional paradigm of public health communication. One might find this communications strategy somewhat paradoxical, but, as we will argue, this conclusion is no longer as obvious if we see the website as part of a wider rhetorical landscape, which is precisely what the Norwegian health authorities did. Ultimately, though, we will argue that *pandemi.no* illustrates the need to use digital media to adjust to the view of expertise that has been emerging in our society—what this website failed to do.

Webs of Experts and Publics

The role of digital media as a means of civic engagement with science and technology has emerged as a favored topic in a wide variety of social science and humanities disciplines (Castells 1996; Beer 2009; Beer and Burrows 2013; Küchler 2008). Likewise, the use of digital media by authorities, including public health officials and organizations, has received increased attention in social studies, public health studies and communication studies (see e.g., Heldman et al. 2013; Thackeray et al. 2012; Neiger et al. 2012; Angeli 2012). As Ruppert and her co-authors have argued, however, theories of how digital media affect the relation between experts and non-experts often seem to lack a certain specificity, as they tend to see digital technologies as forces of "epochal change" (see Ruppert et al. 2013).

In contrast to such sweeping theories, we believe our attempts to understand how digital media rework expert-non-expert relations should be concrete, and that we should pay more serious attention, as Hilgartner argues, to "the techniques, props, and procedures that advisors deploy to build credibility, paying special attention to self-presentation and 'information control'" (Hilgartner 2000: 9). These insights then propose a need to address concrete empirical sites where digital technologies are in use, and pay attention to their productive capacities in specific situations (cf. Ruppert et al. 2013: 28). We need, in other words, to shift our attention to the specificities of digital technologies and study how they generate a new set of circumstances for authority.

By studying a concrete case of how digital platforms and devices are used to communicate and inform in the event of pandemics, we can begin to question ideas of the supposed "epochal change" ushered in by digital media, and instead place into view what Ruppert et al. call the "emerging stabilizations and fixities being performed in cascades of [...] devices in particular locations" (2013: 34). This, they point out, means also to explore how digital devices take part in the making of contemporary sociality (ibid.), which in our case means to explore how the authorities leverage these media in their enactment of themselves *as authorities*.

As noted, one implication of this is that we cannot conceive of authority by means of *ethos* as traditionally understood—where that concept denotes an effort to enact the credibility of the specific speaker in question. Rather, the authorities establish their authority by creating and leveraging the materiality of a specific technology, so that a space is made in and through which they can perform as the proper authorities to speak on the issue at hand. Authority comes, in other words, from a successful combination of rhetoric and materiality, from filling a particular form with the right content. Updating the *ethos* function as a combination of rhetorical creativity and the specific materiality of a particular medium, will allow us to see how authorities reconfigure their expertise in digital media (ibid.: 40). It allows for a view of how the materiality of digital communication technologies entangle with particular rhetorical strategies, to create new forms of address, new types of relations between, say, health authorities and citizens. As importantly, however, it allows us to discover that the hypothesized outcomes of digital media—the "epochal changes"—are *not* always to be found.

Old Mishaps, New Website: *Pandemi.no*

The 2009 pandemic in Norway presents a particularly pertinent case with which to explore these issues, not only because it is the latest pandemic on record and the first one to take place after the advent of the Internet, but because this particular move towards digital media was both deliberate and planned, as part of official preparedness strategies. In line with the Norwegian National Preparedness Plan for Influenza, which had been revised in 2006, the government aimed to ensure the best possible adherence to and results from the governmental measures, through "evidence-based and coordinated information at the right time, on all levels" (HOD 2006: 7). The document introduced a plan for a new website that would have the domain name "pandemi.no." The website was to be activated in the event of a pandemic, to ensure the *efficient* distribution of *consistent* and *evidence-based information*, and was presented as the "main tool" for ongoing broadcasting of information during a pandemic (2006: 26). After the World Health Organization (WHO) declared a pandemic, on 11 June 2009, the web portal went live under the name "Pandemi – Myndighetenes nettside om pandemisk influensa [Pandemic – The Government's Website on Pandemic Flu]."

The website *pandemi.no* was thus part of already existing rhetorical strategies embedded in Norway's preparedness plans. What is particularly noteworthy about these plans is that Norwegian health authorities appeared to have a clear idea of what they wanted to achieve with the website—most notably, that the website could become an alternative to the loud and messy landscape offered by mass media. This idea appeared to have come in part as a response to previous missteps with the media. Prior to the 2009 pandemic, the Norwegian authorities had had several unfortunate encounters with mass media over its response to crises—including the 2004 tsunami and a more recent episode where the estimated number of fatalities from a future pandemic was made front-page news. Top health bureaucrats in the Ministry of Health and Care Services had been working hard to get on top of the situation before the revised version of the preparedness plans appeared in 2006, and *pandemi.no* was one measure they thought could help them avoid the mistakes of the past (see Brekke et al. 2017).

These circumstances on the one hand explain some of the motivations of the Norwegian health authorities, but at the same time, they suggest that the grand story we reproduced above, about digital media being bringers of democratization and symmetrical leveling of expert-non-expert relations, is much too simple. For one, although the mass media demonstrably work under an incentive of public information in cases like this, they never quite let go of another central purpose, namely discussion, debate, and digging for dirt (see Chapter 3 in this volume). Reversely, the effects of digital media do not run in a straight line towards democratization and symmetry. As we will see, *pandemi.no* was a digital medium designed largely to establish authority by retaining some presumably outdated features of the expert-non-expert relation, most notably the assumption that the medical authorities would speak and the public listen.

A Depersonalized Form of Address

Aesthetically as well as technologically, *pandemi.no* is unexceptional, and the first impression one gets is that of an ordinary information website. By this, we mean that when one enters the site, one is presented mainly with text, which is ordered neatly and presumably to allow easy access and overview, and not with any "flashy" design elements or advanced technical features. The website has a white background with turquois font. The title of the website is placed in the upper left corner, below which is a menu bar that leads visitors to subpages titled "Vaccination"; "Limit infection"; "Are you feeling sick?"; "Treatment and medicines"; "Risk groups"; "Questions & Answers"; "Information material"; "Current"; "The Health Sector"; "Advice for Planning"; "Press"; and "Links." The main visual attraction on the website's main page, however, is four turquois-colored boxes entitled "VACCINES," "ILLNESS AND SYMPTOMS," "TREATMENT AND MEDICATION" and "RISK GROUPS." Their graphical presentation immediately invites you to click on one of them, and their visual prominence on the main page would seems to suggest to the visitor four immediate concerns you should have whenever the word "pandemic" comes up. Below these four boxes, there is also a menu bar covering the most recent (and or relevant) news on the pandemic and the Norwegian context.

Turning from the site's visual presentation to the text presented in its web of pages, it becomes clear that each of the tracks a visitor can follow on the site enacts more or less the same version of the relation between experts and non-experts. Overall, that relation is one where a literally impersonal expert speaks to a less-knowing audience. The information and advice on the page does not emanate from an individual expert, presented with, say, name and photo, but rather from an unidentified expert speaker, from a detached voice of science-based advice. The site contains hardly any personal pronouns, whether in singular or plural, images of concrete individuals, or designations of titles, backgrounds, or competencies. This form of presentation stands in clear contrast to the authorities' communication in the mass media, where the three relevant entities of government from day one communicated through three identified spokespersons who—thanks to the frequency of their appearances in the media—quickly became household names. On *pandemi.no*, however, the message is delivered not by any *person*, but by the depersonalized collective voice of expert opinion. This works in concert with a rhetoric that consistently places data, evidence, and cold advice at the center, in an approximation of pure, factual "information."

With a few exceptions, the content provided on the website is not of a technical nature, but accessible to a wide readership, in a mode of popularization. The website assumes a reader which is hungry for information, but which seemingly has no particular leaning in her consumption of it. In other words, the website does not significantly factor in perspectives on the pandemic which are more than a little at odds with the one presented by its own impersonal expert voice. The model user of the website is one who is prone to accept the authority of the health authorities, and who will be further convinced upon meeting the unwavering and uniform advice on *pandemi.no*. Again, this presents us with a contrast to the mass media, where representatives of the health authorities had throughout the pandemic's duration to face challenges to their status and advice, criticisms and debate, and perspectives so at odds with their own that it seemed almost absurd. While the mass media was often a scene of conflict and contestation—not to say a certain communicative chaos (see Bjørkdahl and Carlsen 2017)—the website stuck to a plain and monologic style.

As a whole, it would be no exaggeration to say that *pandemi.no* leverages the materiality of this digital medium to enact a relation between expert and non-expert that, according to the standard story alluded to above, should have been made obsolete by the advent of digital media. To use Collins and Evans' phrase, it seems to have been inconceivable for the makers of *pandemi.no* that advice on the pandemic "could travel in any other direction than from the top down" (2002: 239).

This summary might seem to run counter to our insistence at the start that an act of communication necessarily involves a particular rhetoric in combination with the materiality of a particular medium, for *pandemi. no* might appear to have failed in taking advantage of the materiality of the website as a medium. This would be a misunderstanding, however. Despite the general claims that digital media will lead to democratization and symmetry, etc., it is demonstrably one of the affordances of the website as a medium to enact a hierarchical relation between expert and non-expert, to enact—with both form and content—a relation expert where the former is the maker and keeper of knowledge, and the latter his eager listener. Far from failing to utilize the materiality of the website to establish its authority, *pandemi.no* does precisely that.

Creating a Network of Credibles

To see that this is the case, we can look at the site's use of a central element of this medium, namely hyperlinks. An important aspect of digital communication is of course that it provides opportunities of instant "networking" by way of links. In contrast to analogue texts, where the rather restricted scope of such networking is illustrated by the use of references in reports and scientific publications, digital texts can easily and immediately write itself into a large network of other websites, texts, audio, video, and more.

This was an opportunity that the authorities took advantage of at *pandemi.no*, primarily to establish a network of credible information sources and expertise—assembling, as they themselves describe in the preparedness plan, the necessary and relevant sources of information on the epidemic. This network included the WHO, several (other) entities within the Norwegian health authorities, as well as European expert institutions (like the European Center for Disease Prevention and Control, ECDC). Also attached to this network were official Norwegian information leaflets on epidemic diseases, and ditto on pandemics in different languages. Finally, links forwarded visitors to video and audio material, some of which featured prominent medical scholars from the National Institute of Public Health.

This "network of credibles" provided visitors with even more information than what could be found on the site itself, but that was not all it did. For a start, there appears to be nothing haphazard about this network; rather, it is carefully designed to consolidate further the authority of the voice behind *pandemi.no*. Each node in this network fits criteria that also describe *pandemi.no*: These are all actors that represent a health authority; that speak in a depersonalized and professional tone; and that care more for disseminating "correct information" than for listening to whatever concerns the public might have. In other words, *pandemi.no* places itself into a network of other entities much like itself, and the effect is arguably to consolidate indirectly the authority that the rest of the site establishes more directly. By having its own descriptions and recommendations of the pandemic appear in a much larger network of sites that make much the same descriptions and recommendations, the site suggested that the depersonalized voice on *pandemi.no* was in fact the voice of a long range of institutions, or possibly even of "the health authorities" as such. *Pandemi.no* thus appeared as a showroom that demonstrated the expertise of the health authorities. The great mass of information assembled on the site and in its network left no doubt that the impersonal collective of experts from which the site took its descriptions and recommendations had answers to "every" possible question concerning the pandemic.

Here, we might again note, however, that the website's presentation was somewhat at odds with what went on in other media and contexts. For while the impression one gets from the site is that of *one unified voice*, emanating from an impersonal collective of medical and public health experts, there were actually several cases of medical experts speaking out against the authorities' handling of the pandemic. For one, the two responsible agencies, The Directorate of Health and the Institute of Public Health, did not see eye to eye in every particular; many at the research-oriented Institute felt that the administration-oriented Directorate was taking a too dramatic, too proactive stance (Brekke et al. 2017). Such disagreements within the ranks of medical experts also reached the public sphere on a number of occasions: For example, professor of social medicine, Per Fugelli, wrote an op-ed in August 2009 where he stated that "there are signs that the NIPH and the Directorate are trying to 'crush the rebellion' [people not wanting to get the flu shot] by help of bogeymen, threats and moralizing," and argued that the health authorities should instead take a more "democratic" approach (Fugelli 2009). A professor of medical ethics, Jan Helge Solbakk, told a tabloid newspaper that, "It is crazy to spend this amount of money on a vaccine for the whole of Norway's population" (Lundh 2009), a statement he followed up the year after, when he dubbed the pandemic "one of the biggest medical research scandals in the modern age" (Christensen 2010).

The point here is not necessarily that the critics and skeptics—of which there were quite a few—were right, but that they were neither heard nor acknowledged on *pandemi.no*. The reason they were not, was probably twofold: On the one hand, the health authorities believed they were right and the critics wrong, and while they were willing to engage with critics in the mass media and elsewhere, they had defined *pandemi.no* as a space where they would present their view on the pandemic in a clear, unified voice. This space, if no other, would be one where the authorities could disseminate "correct information." Paradoxically, one might say, they used this new, digital medium to enact a traditional, top-down mode of public health communication that had already become hard to pull off in the mass media.

Seen with a narrow scope, we must acknowledge that *pandemi.no* succeeded in meeting the aim laid down in the Preparedness Plan from 2006, which was to be clear and unambiguous in their communication. While the mass mediation of the pandemic was somewhat schizophrenic and confusing (see Bjørkdahl and Carlsen 2017), the authorities' communication on the site was clear, unequivocal, and steadfast. By keeping the design in an unflashy aesthetic; by using a depersonalized, authoritative form of address; and by assembling a network of credible associations, *pandemi.no* did in fact take advantage of the affordances of the website. They gave the site's user an authoritative account of the threat, as well as a set of unequivocal recommendations about how to meet it. Yet, while the site succeeded in attracting a certain number of the public away from the "messy" mass media, it arguably did not succeed in establishing a dialogue with that public.

Virtual Questions and Answers

For an illustration of this point, we can look more closely at one particular element of the site, which we believe illustrates its general tendency to establish authority in the mode of traditional public health communication. This element is the Q&A section, which one might think is a token of the site-makers' wish to engage the public, to invite them in, as it were, and take steps towards a dialogic mode. Questions and answers are, after all, the stuff of dialogue. This assumption does not hold up, however, as the Q&A in this case rested on much the same assumption about experts and non-experts as the site as a whole.

Clicking on the Q&A link in the menu bar, another page appears which features a new menu bar directing visitors to answers to a range of specific concerns. The total number of questions is sizable, but the range is limited to ten categories: general information on influenza; vaccines; contamination; illness and symptoms; children and influenza; contact with persons with influenza; treatment of ill persons; travel; returning from affected areas; as well as protection and hygiene advice. Clicking on the "vaccines" link, for example, forty-two questions and corresponding answers appear. Questions include "Why vaccinate?," "I have good health, should I vaccinate?," "How is the pandemic vaccine produced?," and "Does the vaccine contain live virus?" The Q&A thus covers general and practical questions as well as some very specific ones. Interestingly, this section, as the site as a whole, touches on many issues that, outside the website, were very controversial, and some of which were the cause of skepticism or criticism of the vaccine.

For instance, questions of how vaccines are produced and of what they contain have historically been and still are crucial concerns for people who are skeptical of vaccines and the vaccine industry. Yet in the Q&A section, the issue is presented as uncontroversial and routine. One answer places vaccine production into a historical continuity: "The vaccine is produced by a traditional, well-tested method, of virus cultivation on eggs." They go on to describe the actual process, including how model vaccines are first made, and how it is tested clinically to ensure satisfactory immune response and safety.

Another example is the question: "Can thiomersal be found in the vaccine?" Presumably, the question speaks to a concern expressed by some members of the public about the content of vaccines, particularly mercury. Here too, though, the answer is framed uncontroversially, by referring to rigorous laboratory work as well as already-established, rigorous practices of vaccine production, concluding that, "Thorough risk assessments of the inclusion of thiomersal have been conducted, a substance which have been used in vaccines for over 70 years. These studies show that thiomersal do not cause health damage."

The same section also includes a question about who is responsible for procuring a pandemic vaccine, to which it answers that the Institute of Public Health, on instructions from the Ministry of Health and Care Services, "in 2008 entered into an agreement with the producer GlaxoSmithKline (GSK) about delivery of a vaccine in the case of a pandemic flu. In total, Norway has an order of 9,4 million doses of pandemic vaccine." Not a word is said to address the concerns that the public and the media had expressed with both aspects of this response, first, that Norway had outsourced vaccine manufacture to a big pharmaceutical company, and second, that Norway—due to its well-off economy—had prioritized access to a surplus of vaccine doses while many poor countries had none at all (Bjørkdahl 2016).

While many of the questions in the Q&A section did gesture to the fact that members of the public might have concerns, this section did not acknowledge that many of those concerns were indeed controversies. The model user of the Q&A was one who simply lacked information, or who might even have heard or read something (e.g., "thiomersal is dangerous") that she was now looking to either confirm or contradict. This model user, however, was already disposed to accept the authorities' authority in the matter. The Q&A never referred to any particular controversy, and it did not address or respond to sources or actors that would have given other answers to the questions listed. The implication throughout was that the health authorities have all the answers worth caring about. By their use of the Q&A, they signaled that they possessed an authority in these questions that other, less credible sources and actors lacked. For instance, they drew on historical evidence and the legitimacy of scientific methods such as laboratory experiments to argue for the safety of the vaccines.

This failure to acknowledge controversy represents, one could say, a reluctance to really engage with the public, and is another example of how the site falls back on a depersonalized form of address. Controversy would threaten this form of address, because one enters a controversy as an identifiable individual, or alternatively institutional, *actor*. But, as we have seen, the premise of *pandemi.no* was precisely the opposite, that a depersonalized collective voice of expert opinion would issue correct information to an obedient and attentive public.

This failure to engage with the public is further underlined by the fact that the Q&A is the closest the website ever gets to an *interactive* feature. Interactivity is, of course, another affordance of the website as a medium, but this was one *pandemi.no* did *not* use. Those visiting the website had no opportunity, for instance, to post comments or add questions of their own. This arguably rendered the website more static and impersonal than it would have been, had a moderator been in place to care for the site and its users. This is somewhat peculiar, as this website was meant to do important health care work in a context of much uncertainty, skepticism, and even controversy. So although the site did include a Q&A, this hardly represented real interactivity. Instead of the public's actual voices, *pandemi.no* provided fictionalized, stylized approximations of them, stripped of any impulse toward disagreement or controversy.

CONCLUSION

Retrospectively, *pandemi.no* can be described as a paradox, perhaps even as somewhat of an anachronism. In the emerging social and cultural landscape, where there was growing skepticism of expertise, and where citizens increasingly were also becoming producers and disseminators of information—not least on digital media—the Norwegian health authorities' website combined rhetoric with material-technological features in a way that recalled the public health communication of times past—a top-down, one-way form of address where expert advice was seen as non-negotiable.

On *pandemi.no*, it was thus as if the status of the scientific expert had never been challenged, as if they need not bother with what Collins and Evans called "the expertise problem." With very few exceptions, the site enacted expertise in a strikingly traditional sense, assuming that when medical authorities spoke, the public would listen. In return, the website did promise to cover everything of relevance, all that the public needed to know. The flipside of this, however, was that they bypassed all critical or controversial opinions or concerns.

For the authorities, *pandemi.no* provided a space away from the "noise" they had come to expect from the media, an opportunity to take control of the message, and fulfill the old dream of disseminating "correct knowledge." In this way, the site did represent one way of taking advantage of this medium's affordances, not to mention that they largely succeeded in executing the directives in the preparedness plans. Successful as this strategy was on its own terms, though, it could of course not make conflict or controversy go away. While the website spoke in a unified and unambiguous—authoritative—voice, it was in fact surrounded by other media where the same issue was often framed as one of contestation and confusion, not to mention one of interests and agendas.

This case should make us reflect on what it should mean to *take advantage of digital media* in preparedness of future pandemics. In one way, the Norwegian authorities did just that during the 2009 pandemic, but, as we have tried to suggest, they did it in a way that did not account for what may be one of the most important features of digital media, namely interactivity—and, more generally, the actual participation of the public. Interactivity/participation is an essential feature to take advantage of, not simply because it is one among the many affordances of digital media, but because this particular one actually responds to the increasing skepticism in our society towards traditional authorities. It is a thus feature with which we could take steps to deal with the "problem of expertise." This would require something more of the health authorities, however, than a willingness to use certain features of a particular medium. It would require a readjustment of their view of themselves and of their relation to the public. For, as one commentator noted in response to the authorities' handling of the 2009 pandemic, "It does not help to be present on Twitter or on television if you deep down think that an open discussion would be unfortunate" (Haug 2009).

REFERENCES

Angeli, Elizabeth. 2012. Metaphors in the Rhetoric of Pandemic Flu: Electronic Media Coverage of H1N1 and Swine Flu. *Journal for Technical Writing and Communication* 42 (3): 203–222.

Beer, David. 2009. Power Through the Algorithm? Participatory Web Cultures and the Technological Unconscious. *New Media and Society* 11 (6): 985–1002.

Beer, David, and Roger Burrows. 2013. Popular Culture, Digital Archives and the New Social Life of Data. *Theory, Culture & Society* 30 (4): 47–71.

Bjørkdahl, Kristian. 2016. Det opplyste opinionsledervelde: Kommentatorstanden under svineinfluensautbruddet i 2009. *Norsk medietidsskrift* 23 (1): 1–22.

Bjørkdahl, Kristian, and Benedicte Carlsen. 2017. Fear of the Fear of the Flu: Assumptions About Media Effects in the 2009 Pandemic. *Science Communication* 39 (3): 358–381.

Brekke, Ole Andreas, Kari Ludvigsen, and Kristian Bjørkdahl. 2017. Handling og usikkerhet: Norske myndigheters kommunikasjon om svineinfluensapandemien i 2009. *Norsk statsvitenskapelig tidsskrift* 33 (1): 54–77.

Castells, Manuel. 1996. *The Information Age: Economy, Society and Culture: Vol. 1. The Rise of the Network Society.* Oxford: Blackwell.

Christensen, Arnfinn. 2010. Vaksine-troverdighet i grus. *forskning.no*, 15 June. https://forskning.no/epidemier-virus-helsepolitikk/vaksine-troverdighet-i-grus/842823.

Collins, Harry, and Robert Evans. 2002. The Third Wave of Science Studies: Studies of Expertise and Experience. *Social Studies of Science* 32 (2): 235–296.

Dosemagen, Shannon, and Lee Aase. 2016. How Social Media Is Shaking Up Public Health and Healthcare. *Huffington Post*, January 27. https://www.huffingtonpost.com/shannon-dosemagen-/how-social-media-is-shaki_b_9090102.html.

Eco, Umberto. 1979. *The Role of the Reader: Explorations in the Semiotics of Texts.* Bloomington: Indiana University Press.

Fugelli, Per. 2009. Vaksinedemokrati. *Verdens Gang* 23 (October): 36.

Gesser-Edelsburg, Anat, and Yaffa Shir-Raz. 2017. *Risk Communication and Infectious Diseases in an Age of Digital Media*. New York: Routledge.

Haug, Charlotte. 2009. … og diskusjoner øker frykten. *Tidsskrift for den norske legeforening* 129 (23): 2469.

Heldman, Amy Burnett, Jessica Schindelar, and James Weaver. 2013. Social Media Engagement and Public Health Communication: Implications for Public Health Organizations Being Truly 'Social'. *Public Health Review* 35 (1): 1–18.

Hilgartner, Stephen. 2000. *Science on Stage: Expert Advice as Public Drama*. Stanford: Stanford University Press.

HOD. 2006. *Nasjonal beredskapslan for pandemisk influensa*. Report from HOD, Norway's Ministry of Health and Care Services. https://www.regjeringen.no/globalassets/upload/kilde/hod/pla/2006/0001/ddd/pdfv/273635-beredskapsplan_pandemi.pdf.

Hutchby, Ian. 2001. Technologies, Texts and Affordances. *Sociology* 35 (2): 441–456.

Jasanoff, Sheila (ed.). 2004. *States of Knowledge: The Co-Production of Science and the Social Order*. London: Routledge.

Küchler, Susanne. 2008. Technological Materiality: Beyond the Dualist Paradigm. *Theory, Culture & Society* 25 (1): 101–120.

Lundh, Francis. 2009. Vanvittig uansvarlig å ikke ha god vaksineavtale. *Verdens Gang*, 7. August. https://www.vg.no/forbruker/helse/i/a5WPL/vanvittig-uansvarlig-aa-ikke-ha-god-vaksineavtale.

Neiger, Brad, Rosemary Thackeray, Sarah Wagenen, Carl Hanson, Joshua West, Michael Barnes, and Michael Fagen. 2012. Use of Social Media in Health Promotion: Purposes, Key Performance Indicators, and Evaluation Metrics. *Health Promotion Practice* 13 (2): 159–164.

Prelli, Lawrence. 1989. *A Rhetoric of Science: Inventing Scientific Discourse*. Columbia: University of South Carolina Press.

Reagle, Joseph. 2015. *Reading the Comments: Likers, Haters, and Manipulators at the Bottom of the Web*. Cambridge: MIT Press.

Ruppert, Evelyn, John Law, and Mike Savage. 2013. Reassembling Social Science Methods: The Challenge of Digital Devices. *Theory, Culture and Society* 30 (4): 22–46.

Shanahan, Marie. 2018. *Journalism, Online Comments, and the Future of Public Discourse*. London: Routledge.

Thackeray, Rosemary, Brad Neiger, Amanda Smith, and Sarah Van Wagenen. 2012. Adoption and Use of Social Media among Public Health Departments. *BMC Public Health* 12: 242.

Wagner-Egger, Pascal, Adrian Bangerter, Ingrid Gilles, Eva Green, David Rigaud, Franciska Krings, Christian Staerklè, and Alain Clemence. 2011. Lay

Perceptions of Collectives at the Outbreak of the H1N1 Epidemic: Heroes, Villains and Victims. *Public Understanding of Science* 20 (4): 461–476.

Wilson, Christopher, and Maria Gabrielsen Jumbert. 2018. The New Informatics of Pandemic Response: Humanitarian Technology, Efficiency, and the Subtle Retreat of National Agency. *Journal of International Humanitarian Action* 3 (8): 1–13.

Xiang, David, Christos Kontos, Afroditi Veloudaki, Agoritsa Baka, Pania Karnaki, and Athena Linos. 2017. Risk Communication in Times of an Epidemic or Pandemic. *Asset Paper Series* 5: 1–14.